"*Keeping Your Boat Afloat When the Big One Hits* is just what the doctor ordered! Kim Hupp provides a powerful prescription for tackling life's challenges before they tackle us. Kim is a living inspiration...and she walks her talk in this inspirational book. It includes a great balance of humorous and creative quotes and anecdotes, thought-provoking questions, and tried-and-true tips and insights for surviving and thriving in life. Drawing on her own personal experience of transforming cancer into a can-do attitude, Kim's empowering spirit is contagious and reflects her beliefs in life-after-birth and life-before-death. *Keeping Your Boat Afloat* will help you add years to your life...and life to your years!"

—*Dr. Joel Goodman, founder and director of The HUMOR Project, Inc. in Saratoga Springs, NY, and author of* Laffirmations: 1,001 Ways to Add Humor to Your Life and Work

"Everyone needs this book. A handbook for surviving the major problems everyone sooner or later will face in life, it is an extraordinary compendium of solutions. Whereas most publications of this sort offer only two or three ways of coping with life, this book is an exhaustive account which includes most of the standard methods developed by others, as well as Kim's own unique and effective strategies. No one could speak to this subject with more authority than does Kimberley Hupp. Assailed many years ago by what appears to be an incurable cancer, and subject to endless surgery and chemotherapy treatments, she always appears in high spirits. A beautiful woman, she looks at least 10 years younger than her actual age. The writing of the book is infused with her buoyant spirit and wonderful sense of humor, that incredible buoyancy by which she kept her own boat afloat. Every page is uplifting, often in delightful and surprising ways. The book is a page-turner, even for those who are fortunate enough at the moment not to need it."

—*James Kettlewell, former Professor of Art at Skidmore College, former curator of the Hyde Collection, and author of the book* Architecture in Saratoga

*(more kind words on the next page...)*

"*Keeping Your Boat Afloat When the Big One Hits* by Kim Hupp is a courageous adventure book, portraying her journey into life's deepest meanings. An often humorous biography, it is nevertheless cram-filled with practical advice and uplifting aphorisms for those suddenly assailed by adversity. Cancer instigated my own inner search, and I found the author's inner revelations cover the gamut of such experiences. A must book for those faced with issues of life or death."
—*David J. Pitkin, author of* Spiritual Numerology: Caring for Number One

"What a precious gift Kim has given to us all! No one can read this book and not be touched by her beautiful spirit, sense of humor, determination, and courage. Not only is Kim a role model for how to approach obstacles in our lives, but she has also given us lots of practical information to help us navigate our own white water experiences. This is a "must read" for anyone who plans on living beyond tomorrow!"
—*Barbara Glanz, CSP, author of* CARE Packages for the Workplace, CARE Packages for the Home, *and* Handle with CARE

"*Keeping Your Boat Afloat When the Big One Hits* is a first-person account of someone who has been there and done that. It was such a joy to read a manuscript where the person's heart is right there on the page. Kim's story is incredibly moving. I admire her courage and strength and am so glad she is sharing her story with others. I believe it will really make a difference for anyone who has the pleasure and privilege of reading this book."
—*Sam Horn, author of* ConZentrate *and* What's Holding You Back?

"An empowering and remarkable book. It is chock full of practical user-friendly steps to help promote the healing process. A must read."
—*Margie Levine, author of* Surviving Cancer

# Keeping Your Boat Afloat
# When the **Big** One Hits

### A practical crisis survival guide

## Kim Hupp

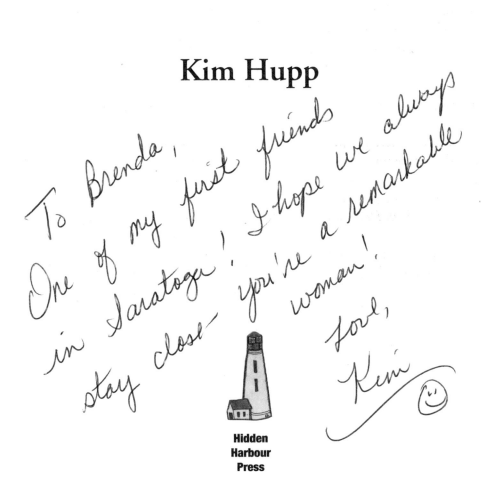

To Brenda,
One of my first friends
in Saratoga, I hope we always
stay close — you're a remarkable
woman!
love,
Kim

**Hidden**
**Harbour**
**Press**

KEEPING YOUR BOAT AFLOAT WHEN THE BIG ONE HITS
KIM HUPP

Published by Hidden Harbour Press
P.O. Box 789
Saratoga Springs, NY 12866

Design and production by Rich Text & Graphics, Saratoga Springs, NY
Copy editing by Gwen Guarino
Cover and author photo by Elizabeth Callen
Printed by A&M Printers, Cambridge, NY

Library of Congress Control Number: 2002112707
ISBN: 0-9723724-0-7

Many of the quotes used in this book were provided by friends of the author,
or were found on the Internet. If you are the author of any unattributed quote,
please write to the above address and we will credit you in any future edition.

# Acknowledgments

A sincere and heartfelt thank you goes to the many people who helped me along the way while writing this book. Without all of you, I could never have done it. I would like to thank Jim and Cindy Loman who helped me come up with such a great title; Richard Romano, who helped with content editing and the technical aspects; my sister, Karen Hupp, who helped in countless ways; and my mother, Dorothy F. Hupp, whose monetary support was invaluable. Thanks also to Dean Waters for the wave.

I would like to thank the Black Crow Network, and the late Vaughn Ward for teaching me about the nuts and bolts of getting a book published, and to David Pitkin for his help in the publishing world of which I knew so little.

Finally, I would like to thank my children, Jessica and Elizabeth Callen, who are the heart and soul of my life, and who are the real heroes in this story. Without them, I would not have had the inspiration, dedication, and will to survive all the traumatic events in my life.

# Table of Contents

### What I Believe

1. I believe there is an intelligence greater than me.
2. I believe if you have the will and the desire to do something, you can.
3. I believe it's important to have a reason to do the thing you want to do.
4. I believe it's important to have role models to follow and supporters to give you the strength to follow them.
5. I believe it is vital to feed your soul its heart's desire.
6. I believe my body will tell me what it needs if only I will listen.
7. I believe God gives us only what we can handle, but will give us challenges to help us grow.
8. I believe that love is the greatest power, the greatest healer, and the greatest gift we could ever give or receive.
9. I believe in miracles.

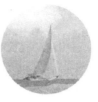

# Introduction
## Keeping Your Boat Afloat

When the doctor told me nine years and four recurrences later that my breast cancer had traveled into my liver, I knew I not only needed to follow the ideas in this book, I needed a miracle. God has given me one. I am alive today by the grace of God and the knowledge of my doctors and care givers, and sane because I used the concepts I have given to you in this book. Living with cancer is difficult at best, and continuing treatment as a single parent in a new location with no base support group was mind boggling. So many people ask me, "How do you do it?" One particularly trying morning I listed everything I had done to not only keep me going, but help me deal with a life threatening disease, moving to a new location with teen-agers, living on my own as a single parent, and making new friends. Thus the idea for this book was born.

So many people have helped me along my "cancer journey" and I am eternally grateful to all of you. When I hear the term "earth angels," I think of you. People also ask me where I get the strength to keep going, even in the face of what some falsely believe is my impending death, according to the statistics. I believe my strength comes from an inner well of faith, hope, and love. I believe God is at the core of that well, and when I have reached bottom and feel I can no longer continue, I feel a warmth and love gurgling up within me that I know is not originating in my being. I also believe some of my strength comes from my family—a long line of stubborn, obstinate, tenacious, "rough, tough, mean, and ornery" folk. During my "growing up years" my family was difficult at best and abusive at worst, but thanks to them I developed a tough, resilient spirit, similar to the pioneers who took on the elements and the dangers of traveling "out west."

I never believed the statistics. I refused to give up even when I had reached bottom and had absolutely nothing left. I decided my own prognosis. "I'm going to live a good long life." My doctors contributed to my conviction to stay alive. They said, "Yes, your cancer is extensive, but you're going to be all right." They never gave me depressing lectures, just a "can do" attitude. This is what is going on, and this is what we're going to do about it. That is exactly the attitude I needed from them.

I believe we have the ability to stare death in the face, eyeball to eyeball, and say, (quaking at first, then with conviction,) "It's not my time to go. I am going to stay here on earth until I have finished what it is I came here to do. Leave me now and come back some other day when I am ready for you."

I also believe we get back what we give out. You may have heard the adage, "You reap what you sow." Being a backyard gardener, I love this saying, and try to live every day sowing love, peace, and caring. I know when I got sick, people came from everywhere to help me; people I didn't even really know very well. They inevitably said something like, "I remember the day you helped me carry my groceries," or "You gave me the nicest smile on a day I really needed it." Kindness is contagious, and I spread as much of it as I can.

I thank all of you who have been praying for me for so long. I am eternally grateful to you for your prayers and support. Without them, I could never have made it.

Happiness can be possible, even during the most troubling times, if you follow this formula my sister's friend gave me: When you get up in the morning, you must have something to do, someone to love, and something to look forward to. I tried to follow this advice during my cancer treatments and found that it really works. My cancer journey was horrifying, difficult, wearying, and long, but because of it I have found happiness, peace, and a deeper understanding of people, life, and the reason we are all here.

I have been told that I am an inspiration because of my positive outlook on life, my unquenchable, happy spirit, and my refusal to give up. My sister wrote me the day I told her about the liver metastases. I told her I was OK, not afraid, but tired and discouraged. I had been fighting cancer for nine years, and it had become such a part of my life that it seemed normal. Maybe I needed to get to that point so I wasn't afraid any more. During those nine years I had undergone surgeries too numerous to count or remember, three separate chemo treatments, radiation, reconstructive surgery, a bone marrow transplant, three different hormone treatments, and side effects I have chosen to forget.

My sister wrote a letter to me and said, "I understand the part about you feeling discouraged, and you're entitled, of course. I allowed myself ten minutes yesterday to be scared, discouraged, and upset. Then I refused to give in any more, because I see now more than ever how fear, discouragement, and hopelessness eat away at our healing and recuperative powers. I believe your simple insistence not to give in to this is what has kept you going all this time. The people who love you get strength from you and your strength. And then when we are strong, you get strong because the people around you are positive and not afraid. I really believe those negative feelings become contagious; it's the fear that does us in! I have said prayers thanking God for your strength because the world needs to hear from you."

I also believe this quote: "The people on our planet are not standing in a line single file. Look closely. Everyone is really standing in a circle, holding hands. Whatever you give to the person standing next to you eventually comes back to you." I have tried to live my life doing good things for people, yet taking care of myself at the same time. This requires a delicate balance. Once we find it, our lives will change for the better. The good things we do for others will come back to us, and we will find the peace and happiness we yearn for.

The beginning of each chapter lists several questions for you to ponder as you read it. I have added funny quotes and anecdotes to help illustrate my point. Cancer and crises are certainly not funny, but if we can find the humor in any situation, it helps lighten things up and bring us to a place we can better deal with it.

I have received gifts too numerous to count from so many people and I thank you from the bottom of my heart. My gift back to you is this book. I hope you will find it helpful for keeping your boat afloat when the big one hits!

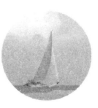

# Eat, Drink, and Be Merry

## Practice Good Nutrition

*Everything I like is either illegal,*
*immoral, or fattening.*

—*Alexander Woollcott*

How carefully do you watch what you eat? Do any of the following apply to you?

- I am at my ideal weight.
- I know what "healthy food" is, even if I don't always eat it.
- I make it a point to always eat healthy food.
- I generally eat healthy, although ice cream occasionally beckons.
- I read the labels on all the processed food I buy.
- I know what all the ingredients are in the foods I eat.
- I like myself just as I am right now.
- I know a healthy way to lose weight.
- I insist that chocolate is one of the four major food groups.

If you answered false to any of the above, you're certainly not alone. Let's face it, we all *know* what foods are healthy and what we *should* be eating, but bad food is just so darn *good!* Why good nutrition is important is no mystery, but it's especially important for crisis management. (As for the last choice above—as unfair as it may seem, no, chocolate is not a major food group!)

**Turkey Day**

> *Excess on occasion is exhilarating.*
> *It prevents moderation from acquiring*
> *the deadening effect of a habit.*
>
> —*W. Somerset Maugham*

W aves of mouth-watering roasting turkey aromas wafted up the stairs into my bedroom. The turkey had been cooking since 6:00 A.M. and I had crawled back to bed for a few extra winks. Twenty hungry guests were coming for dinner in a few hours, and there was still much to be done. Thanksgiving was always my holiday. I enjoyed cooking and preparing for this great feast that brought family and friends together. And what a feast! Sage-roasted turkey with caramelized onions, mashed potatoes with gravy, creamed onions with mushrooms and carrots, yams drizzled with marshmallow. Warm cranberry bread, old-fashioned pumpkin pie, cinnamon-spiced apple pie and hot mulled cider. Mixed nuts and green olives, cheese and crackers, and Australian Chardonnay. Traditions handed down and collected throughout the years still bring us together for a time of feasting and fun.

Associations with food, traditions and holidays are strong. What's the first thing we think of when we think of a holiday? Most of the time it's the type of food associated with it. What are some of your favorite memories of traditions and food? In New England on a crisp fall Saturday in October, after raking and burning leaves, nothing was better than Boston baked beans, hot dogs, brown bread and cider. The smell of burnt leaves lingering on our clothes, the joy of jumping in giant leaf piles, rolling around and tossing them into the air, and breathing in the rich, pungent earth smells fills me with happy contented childhood memories. One of my favorite memories is smelling the Yankee pot roast and Yorkshire pudding with roasted potatoes coming from the kitchen when I returned from church late on Sunday mornings. Whatever happened to a good, old-fashioned Sunday dinner with all of the family gathered around a table set with the best china and crystal and serving dishes of Grandma's best meatloaf and mashed potatoes?

Food is synonymous with celebrations. Weddings, graduations, job promotions, house parties, sports events, meetings—just about any time people get together socially wouldn't be as much fun without food. What would a Superbowl game be without beer, nachos, and cheese? Who wouldn't serve wine, cheese, and crackers at a house party? What would a banquet be without tempting appetizers and rich gooey desserts? And isn't the most prominent object at a wedding reception the towering wedding cake? Food and social situations go hand in hand.

And it's not just us food-loving Americans. Just about every culture on Earth—past and present—associates food with social occasions. It may very well be a fundamental part of human nature. And given that aspect of human nature, you can see what we're up against when it comes to nutrition.

What constitutes good nutrition? What is healthy food? Who's eating it? Ask any 10 people about nutrition, healthy eating, and food, and you'll get 10 different answers. There are those who swear by a vegetarian diet, while others have to have their meat and potatoes. Diets can be as varied as macrobiotic, live food, raw food, juice diets, blood-type diets, vegan diets, and Weight Watchers. A balanced diet to one person might mean adding a salad to a burger and fries while to another it might mean eating textured vegetable protein and a fruit compote. It seems like every week some new medical report comes out that refutes the findings of an earlier report. Salt is bad. No, wait, this week salt is good. Wouldn't it be ironic if we find out 200 years from now that ice cream, desserts, and burgers were the healthiest things after all?

Then there are those who mix diet and politics—any food that comes from an animal is bad, or food that kills plants is bad (i.e., those who only eat fruit). There is so much confusion, contradictory information, and charged emotion that it's enough to make anyone throw up their hands in exasperation and grab another bag of M&Ms.

Obviously we need food to stay alive, but there is more to it than just that. In cultures where food is scarce, people eat to survive. In other cultures where food is plentiful, it co-exists with joy and celebration. Food influences our health and well being. It provides pleasure and comfort, especially when we are sick or unhappy. Remember mom's chicken soup when you were sick and the "mother of all comfort foods"—macaroni and cheese—when you were feeling blue? Food supplies the basic needs of the body for calories and nutrients, it can either reduce or enhance risk of disease, and it can fortify our immune system for healing.

We get our information about food from registered dietitians, government agencies, physicians, nurses, alternative practitioners, food technologists, bookstores, TV, newspapers, magazines, health food stores, and the Internet. Most of the information is contradictory, some of it is unscientific, and many times it is intended to promote a new product or supplement, or even a political viewpoint.

**You Are What You Eat**

*If you are what you eat,*
*don't be a four-day-old burrito.*

—*Quote from a food magazine*

When my cancer returned for the fourth time, I began to investigate the possibility that what I ate might help or hurt me. My oncologist told me to just "eat a balanced diet" which basically consisted of the USDA's food pyramid. I knew all about food groups and so on, but I wanted more information. What kind of flour should I use—whole wheat or white? What type of cooking oil—olive or canola? I wanted more specifics. What about pesticides? Does eating organic really lower our cancer risk? Should we use the vegetable wash sold in the supermarkets to rinse off the pesticides or will ordinary dish detergent do just as well at half the cost? What I found was mountains of information, mostly conflicting, that ultimately confused me all the more.

My mean old English grandmother, Grandma Floyd, for all her faults, was way ahead of her time as far as her philosophy on nutrition. Her recommendation for a healthy diet was short and sweet: "Eat your greens for a good bowel movement," and "Anything in moderation." She used corn oil margarine, ate a soft-boiled egg every morning, drank English tea with her friend every afternoon, ate meat and potatoes, bacon and gravy, and had a nip of red wine every night for her iron-poor blood ("doctor's orders"). She lived well, was hearty and active, ate her greens and anything in moderation, and lived to be 90 years old. You probably have a relative with a similar approach to diet (or lack thereof) who could boast a similar longevity. Anecdotal evidence is not science, but it does throw a monkey wrench into what we think of as healthy living and the advantages it's supposed to have.

Basically, it's all a question of attitudes toward food—and there are more of them than you'd think.

Food has become a huge industry. This is where the confusion comes in. When there is money to be made, there is something to protect. Big corporations use the media to spread information to promote their particular products. That's what advertising is, after all. But just because something is advertised to us doesn't mean that it's necessarily good for us. (This is likely why few advertisers of food products even mention nutrition—if you watch food commercials it's all about "yumminess," convenience, or even lifestyle.) It is up to us, if we want to practice good nutrition, to take the time to sift through the information we're bombarded with, decide what is true and helpful and what is simply advertising, and make our own choices about what we eat. The harder someone pushes an idea, the more we should investigate it. What's in it for me? What's in it for them?

Eating is a major source of pleasure, so we must be careful about what we eat and how often we eat it. The appearance and the smell of food along with the taste and feel in the mouth create a wonderful, pleasurable experience, as well as a satisfying feeling of being nourished. When these pleasurable sensations are combined with good company, uplifting music and a festive atmosphere, it can do wonders for our health and well-being. Isn't it one of the best experiences in the world to be at a fantastic party with wonderful friends eating delicious food, listening to fabulous music and having a spectacular time?

**Feast Not Famine**

> *I am not a glutton. I am an explorer of food.*
> —Erma Bombeck

Bunratty Castle in County Clare, Ireland, built in 1425, is the setting for tourists to enjoy Medieval banquets. My daughters and I were lucky enough to attend one of the "Earl of Thomond's" special banquets, replete with fiery torches blazing greetings up the curved stone steps to the castle, bright, cheery banners bearing the Earl's coat of arms, winsome maidens in red and blue velvet strumming harps and violins, and a cup of mead for each guest. Sitting down at huge wooden banquet tables, we were served by lovely maidens and handsome lads. We slurped our hearty steaming soup right from the bowls, just as they did hundreds of years ago. We stabbed large pieces of meat and potatoes with thick knives (evidently forks had not been invented during that time) pulling the meat off ever so carefully so as not to cut ourselves, and wiped our plates clean with dark grained bread. Huge trays that held delicious desserts that replenished again and again. Continuous refills of cups of mead kept us in continuous good spirits. Laughter, warmth, and fun filled us all with sensual pleasures that were not soon forgotten! Guests young and old shared a bond during that evening of fun and food and song and drink.

The food we ate that night (and the staggering amounts of it!) may not have been on the dieter's acceptable foods list, but the good will and good spirits that accompanied it made it all right. As this was a one-time feast and not a nightly orgy of food, we did not suffer any ill effects from all the merriment. If we ate like this night after night, surely our doctors and our cholesterol would be screaming, "Enough!" Eating is an important part of social interaction, but too much of a good thing is not such a good thing. Eating and drinking to excess will make anyone sick; our bodies simply cannot tolerate that kind of abuse. Remember Grandma Floyd's admonition, "Anything in moderation."

## Bubble and Squeak and Finnan Haddie

*The first thing I remember liking
that liked me back was food.*
—*Rhoda Morgenstern Gerard (from the TV show Rhoda)*

Food also defines and reflects our cultural identity. While lunching with a friend at a trendy gourmet restaurant in Siesta Key, Florida, I noticed bubble and squeak, finnan haddie, steak and kidney pie, and Yorkshire pudding on the menu. Because I had grown up eating this food with the curious names, I knew the owner must be English. I looked around to ask the waitress and noticed several pictures of Queen Elizabeth, Princess Diana and Prince Charles, and walls covered with lovely scenes of English gardens. The owner came out to speak to us, and her accent confirmed my suspicions. If I had seen codfish cakes, pork and clams, Sintra cheesecakes, or caldo verde, I would have suspected the owner to be Portuguese.

People's diets generally revolve around the geographic area they live in. If a group of people settles near the ocean, much of the local cuisine will come from the sea. Cooking practices also reflect different cultures. When I lived in Lisbon, Portugal, in the 1970s, lunchtime was a special treat for me. I loved walking along the cobbled sidewalks of the city smelling the delicious aroma of freshly caught sardines sizzling on small hibachis right on the sidewalks! It's a custom I hope is still being practiced today.

Fish and chips has always been one of my favorite meals, and the size of the fish portions near the New England coast where I grew up was large and plentiful. The fish was usually coated with a delicious crispy batter. When I ordered fish and chips in New York City, my friend warned me it would be a little different from what I was used to, and she was right—the fish was small, dried up, and breaded. When I'm in the Southeastern United States I always eat lots of exotic tropical fruit that I can't get fresh when I am up North. Southwestern food is usually served with some zing and pizzazz to it, and my mother once told me this was because in the "olden days" they had to add spice to the food to hide the taste of spoilage. Whatever the reason, it sure tastes good! Because our food is so closely tied with culture, family traditions and customs, there is a tremendous psychological, social and cultural investment involved in our eating patterns. If we must change our diets for health reasons, there is a lot more to change than just the food.

## High-Octane Food

> *The only way to keep your health is to eat*
> *what you don't want, drink what you*
> *don't like, and do what you'd rather not.*
>
> —*Mark Twain*

Food is just one part of what determines our health. Genetics plays a large role as do environmental, psychosocial, and spiritual aspects. Several other factors are important to our health: the type and amount of exercise we get; sources of stress in our lives and how we deal with that stress; sources of strength such as religion, spirituality, and our community of supportive friends; getting enough sleep; our relationships with spouses, children, parents, friends, and co-workers; whether or not we take food supplements, or drink coffee or alcohol; and any past illnesses. Food is but one part of a very complex set of rules that govern our bodies, yet it is significant. Our bodies are really energy systems that function optimally with the correct fuel. The analogy of putting cheap gas in your car is a good one. I am in the process of selling my gas-guzzling SUV. When gas prices rise, I put the lowest octane gas in it. Consequently, I get engine knocks, I can't use the cruise control because there is not enough power, and it takes a much greater effort to climb hills. So it is with our bodies. If we put in non-nutritious food, we get less energy, complaints from our stomachs and other organs, and generally not as much mileage out of our bodies as we could if we ate healthier food.

Since we can choose what we put in our mouths, we must realize that the responsibility for good health is ours. So, without feeling guilty, anxious or uncomfortable, how can we practice good nutrition in a culture that encourages us to eat unhealthy food, and lots of it?

Let's first look at what has happened to our food over the past century. Our food has changed drastically in the last few decades by the addition of pesticides, additives, preservatives, artificial flavorings and colorings, dehydration, concentration, genetic modification, freezing, canning, microwaving, irradiation, and growth hormones. Cows and chickens are raised in crowded conditions that promote infections. Antibiotics are given to fight the infections, and these antibiotics stay in the meat and end up in our bodies. Fish that are farmed do not have as many minerals and nutrients as those from the deep ocean fishing grounds, and fish that is caught fresh has all the vitamins and minerals, but may come from polluted waters.

When I lived in Portugal I was invited to a "Festa da Vinho Verde," or New Wine Feast. After the grapes have been harvested and properly stomped on, put through the press, and the wine is aged and finally ready to drink, there is a grand celebration complete with a parade through the streets of town; loud, happy music; children banging pots and pans; huge amounts of all types of food; and, of course, freely flowing wine. A few friends and I gathered at a neighbor's home to share in the festivities. A gigantic platter of pork and clams filled the table, along with Portuguese sweet bread, caldo verde soup, watercress salad and *arroz doce* (sweet rice) for dessert. As I savored every tantalizing mouthful, I could smell the tangy salt water of the beach close by. Joyfully, our host informed us the clams we were eating were from the very same beach we could see beyond the house. Horrified, I almost choked on my next bite. The waters of the Estoril beach were extremely polluted, but there was no health department to close it down! Villagers blissfully ate the fish from the polluted waters unaware of the diseases waiting to sicken them. We prayed to the gods of the new wine to save us from food poisoning, hepatitis, or worse. We were lucky and stayed well. To this day I will not eat shellfish unless I know where it came from and that it has been cooked to within an inch of its life.

Unfortunately many pollutants are allowed in fish under guidelines determined by the government. The public has a right to know if the fish they're eating has "acceptable" levels of pollutants. It's frightening to think that someone I don't know is deciding for my body what is an acceptable level of poison. How can they tell the difference for a 200 pound man and a 125 pound woman? It would be better if we did not have to worry about pollutants at all.

Some common complaints that can be traced to the food we eat are: being overweight and obese, coronary artery disease, high blood pressure, cancer, ulcers, backaches, migraine headaches, arthritis, and strokes. If we know we are getting sick from our food, and studies show that indeed this is true, why are we not doing more to eat better? Perhaps it's because it takes too much effort to learn about healthy eating and to change our eating patterns. Perhaps it's because of the traditions and culture surrounding the type of food we eat. Yet it's much easier than you think. Check out one of the newer grocery stores. There are huge sections of "natural" food, organic food, and even packaged fresh dinners. Today as I was shopping I noticed a "weekend dinners" section of the market offering fresh meatloaf with ketchup, a container of mashed potatoes, grilled chicken teriyaki with rice, pizza bagels with pepperoni and cheese, and baked noodles with sour cream. They looked delicious, were affordable, were much healthier than fast food (yet could be technically called "fast food"), and convenient. A young man was checking it out, and I thought it was absolutely perfect for a single career person who simply does not have the time to cook from scratch. Let your friendly grocer do it for you!

### Arame, Kombu, Mochi, Umeboshi: What the Heck Is That?
*When in doubt, eat a plant.*

—*Greg Anderson*

When I began studying diet and cancer, I thought I might try a macrobiotic diet. The Kushi Institute in Massachusetts claimed miraculous cures using its diet. It seemed like a much better idea to eat good food and get rid of cancer than undergo chemotherapy again, but when I researched the diet it was a bit overwhelming. Just learning new words such as arame (a black sea vegetable), kombu (a dark green sea vegetable), mochi (a cake made from cooked, pounded sweet rice), and umeboshi (a salted pickled plum paste used as a seasoning) was daunting. Now I had to learn where to find them, be able to identify them, learn how to cook them, and hope I would like them. It didn't work. It was too difficult for me to switch to a completely different diet. I had too many strong traditions, emotions, and social connections related to the food I ate and eating a strictly Japanese diet filled me with despair. I realized that if the diet were too rigid, it could become a form of self-punishment that would cause negative feelings, and this is completely against the diet's principles. I chose instead to use some of the ingredients and try to adapt some of the practices into my lifestyle. I liked the idea of being in a positive frame of mind while cooking, and everyone wants to know my secret ingredient for my now famous butternut squash soup. (Add a tablespoon or so of umeboshi paste.)

### Pass the Biggie Fries, Please
*Part of the secret of success in life is to eat what you like and let the food fight it out inside.*

—*Mark Twain*

As a nation, Americans tend to be overweight. Sitting at the airport in Sarasota, Florida, waiting for my flight home, I studied the passengers boarding the plane. It surprised me to see how many people could be considered overweight. Why is this so? Partly because we have so much food, partly because of the food industry, and partly because we may use food to fulfill other needs. Medication, cancer treatment, or hormonal problems contribute to some of our problems with weight, and some people simply have slower metabolisms than others. As a general rule though, many of us would like to shed a few pounds.

There are other factors that may cause us to eat. How many times have you eaten something because you were bored, tired, anxious, lonely, angry, feeling unloved or unfulfilled? If we could work on those areas of our lives that are being neglected instead of using food to "fix" them, we could eliminate a lot of extra calories from our daily dose!

One of the worst outcomes of our busy lifestyles has been the fast-food industry. One meal at a fast food restaurant can use up a whole day's worth of calories! We have traded convenience, familiarity, and time for food that may be literally killing us. Some of the worst food we could ever possibly eat comes from fast-food chains. We would do better buying a prepared sandwich from the grocery store or even skipping lunch altogether. Toys and play centers entice the younger ones into these places, and large monetary donations for cancer research and care promote good will in the community, successfully switching our focus from the "bad" food, to the "good intentions" of the corporate fast-food giants.

Another reason we're getting larger as a population is that we are also getting larger helpings. Most restaurants now serve a portion of food that normally would feed three. We see mega-muffins, mega cookies, and mega sizes in warehouse stores, big burgers, biggie fries, quarter pounders, and super sizes. All-you-can-eat buffets are becoming popular again, but they promote overindulgence. I find it particularly difficult to say no to a second helping of sweet-and-sour chicken, pork fried rice, and shrimp lo mein at my favorite Chinese restaurant even when I feel somewhat full! I have learned to stay away from the buffet and order instead from the menu. The food is fresher and I can do without the second helping.

How can we manage our hunger, tame those temptations, control our appetites, forsake the sin of gluttony and eat better and safer with all of this working against us? It won't be easy, but we can begin by becoming aware of the problem, learning as much as we can about it, and using the information we have to make better choices about the food we eat. This does take some time and effort, but if you truly want to look better, feel better, and live longer, it's worth the work. And keep your sense of humor about the whole thing. As George Carlin says, "If you try to fail and succeed, which have you done?"

## Thought for Food

The nuts and bolts of healthy eating for me are:

- eat more fruits and vegetables
- avoid processed food
- buy organic
- cook from scratch whenever possible
- cut down on fat, red meat and dairy products,
- drink more fresh well water (but not necessarily eight glasses a day)
- cut down on caffeine, sugar and alcohol
- eat in moderation (of course!)

Do I practice all of these all the time with laserlike focus? Of course not. I know that I should probably use less butter, but I like it too much. I cut out fat in other areas so I can eat butter to my heart's content. It's important for you to make your own decisions about what you eat, and be aware of the consequences of your diet. Try to balance a "bad" food with some healthier ones so you can continue to eat some of the foods you like. Healthy eating doesn't have to mean complete sacrifice of any enjoyment from food.

### The Decadent Chocolate Bar

*Take time to deliberate, but when the time*
*for action arrives, stop thinking and go in.*

—*Andrew Jackson*

I am a true chocoholic, and will never forget the chocolate bar at the top of the Hyatt Regency in New Orleans. Yes, New Orleans is a decadent city, and whatever your weakness may be, they will provide for it. Mine happens to be chocolate. I was in chocolate heaven when I saw that bar. My mouth started watering before I even saw what was there. I stared longingly atayered chocolate cake with fudge frosting, chocolate mousse covered with whipped cream, white chocolate candy, dark chocolate truffles, milk chocolate kisses and confections, mint chocolate chip cookies, French chocolate pudding, and more than I could ever remember or eat! But what a night! For the next three days I was as good as gold with my diet, and it was worth every savory, decadent delicious bite.

Decide how you will eat healthier, but have fun with it. The goal in life is to be happy and healthy, not hung up on what we are eating. Of course, if you are on a strict diet for coronary heart disease or any other ailment, listen to your doctor, not me! Common sense is the rule here.

One of the best books I have read on diet and good nutrition is "Eating Well for Optimum Health" by Andrew Weil, M.D., published by Alfred Knopf. He has researched data and has sound scientific answers to most questions regarding good nutrition. He details fats, proteins, carbohydrates, vitamins, and minerals and how they affect our general health. He discusses how to make decisions about the latest miracle diet or reducing aid, and he gives an optimum diet with recipes and nutrition breakdowns. He has a common-sense approach to diet that I found refreshing.

Caution should be heeded when researching supplements and diet products. A dear friend of mine told me about a pill that would absolutely cure cancer. He brought over a magazine-type newsletter with a cover splashed with huge red letters that read, "READ THIS OR DIE!" The entire newsletter boasted the healing powers of these pills, how they were the cure for cancer, and were so cutting edge that this doctor was the only one who knew about them. Immediately I was suspicious, but I called the toll-free number. I couldn't order the pills unless I became a member of the newsletter that would cost only $50.00 a year. Does this sound a little suspicious to you? It sure did to me. I didn't order the pills.

Remember, if something sounds too good to be true, it probably is. If there really were a diet or magic pill that could cure cancer or make us lose weight without cutting down on our food intake, we would all know about it. Question every statement you read. Ask for solid proof. Ask who is writing the article. Who is the publisher, and why are they so motivated to sell this particular product? Snake oil is alive and well in the 21st century. Buyer beware.

Should we diet if we are overweight? It's my personal belief that most "fad" diets just don't work. When you're dieting, what is your constant focus? Food! It's all you can think about. Your day revolves around what you are not going to eat today, and this leads to a feeling of deprivation. Feeling deprived causes you to want the restricted food all the more. Being on a regimented diet for a long period of time is just too difficult for most people, especially when it conflicts with our old patterns of eating. Usually we stop dieting once we have lost the desired weight, and go back to our original eating patterns. Most of us gain back the weight it took us so long to lose, and end up feeling guilty, depressed, demoralized and fat again.

A better way to lose weight is to change our present patterns of eating. This will usually include lifestyle changes. If you have a health threatening weight gain you need to do something serious about it, and may have to seek help from a professional. But if you are leading a relatively active and healthy lifestyle, eating well and exercising, you may be fine just the way you are. If you really want to lose some weight there are some better ways to do it than by dieting (which are listed at the end of this chapter).

Remember that skinny was not always considered attractive. (In prior centuries, being overweight was a status symbol—a sign that you had money and could afford to eat a lot.) Miniskirts and mini sizes (in bodies, not food) ushered in the age of Aquarius and the likes of the British model "Twiggy" in the early 1970s. This helped set the stage for our present compulsion for skin and bones. The models on the cover of the glamour magazines today look like sick, pale skeletons draped in fancy fabric. Many women and men have had plastic surgery to "correct" problems with their bodies, including surgery to remove ribs to make their stomachs smaller. Tummy tucks are commonplace, as is liposuction.

Most of us have bought into at least some of the corporate clatter, myself included, but now we can arm ourselves against the assault to our egos, and claim our bodies to be beautiful just as they are. An affirmation to repeat every morning might be, "I accept and love myself just as I am. I do not have to look like the corporate image of what 'beautiful' is." When looking at pictures of supermodels, just remember that anyone can look beautiful in pictures if you airbrush out all the defects.

**You're Fine Just the Way You Are Now**
Physicians love to lump us all together with tables, charts, and numbers, and some of those charts may cause you to feel that you are over- or underweight when in fact you're perfectly fine. I find it wrong to lump everybody in one category without taking into consideration anything else about that person. My daughters' pediatrician loved to quote numbers and charts and graphs when examining my babies, and I used to drive him crazy when I poo-pooed it all. I could see him cringe when I said, "Their cheeks are rosy, they have lots of cute baby fat, they're smiling and full of life, and I don't need any numbers or charts or graphs to tell me they are healthy!" Needless to say, my children's doctor did not smile whenever he saw my name on the appointment list.

Take into consideration all the factors about you that might put you in a different weight table. Don't believe everything you read or be too rigid about what you believe to be true.

You may not like yourself at your present weight. If you feel that you want to lose a little weight, remember you are perfect just the way you are right now. Love yourself wholly and affirm, "I love myself just as I am. There are some things I would like to change about myself, such as losing a little weight, but this will not make me a better person. I am fine just as I am." Begin your plan for losing weight and congratulate yourself that you are making some positive changes in your life. Always make any life changes a positive experience so they will become permanent. If you berate yourself or make yourself wrong, why would you want those changes to be lasting? Loving yourself through all of the changes is the most important thing you can do for yourself.

### Don't Shop When You're Hungry

*I tried to save grocery money once, but some of the suggestions were just not practical; like "Don't shop when you're hungry," which eliminated all hours when the store was open.*

—Erma Bombeck

Experiment with different ways to manage your hunger when you are trying to lose weight. Drinking a large glass of water before and after each meal fills you up quite nicely. If you are going to a banquet or holiday feast where there will be tables of tempting food and drink, eat some healthy food before you go to the party. That way you will be less hungry when you arrive, and you'll have control over what you eat. Join in with the crowd, eat what you want, and have fun. You'll leave the party feeling a lot happier, and with much less guilt than if you had come ravenously hungry and eaten everything in sight.

Another way to manage hunger is to eat several small meals during the day instead of the usual three. Drink a large glass of water and have a small healthy snack between meals. Find out what works for you. Remember that counting calories and feeling deprived will probably not work. Eating with abandon will not work either. There must be a healthy balance between the two. A good affirmation to begin each day might be: "I can eat anything and everything I want today. I choose to eat this particular food today, this amount of food, and will feel healthy and happy because I chose wisely."

**Stay Away From Mrs. London's! (But only if you're dieting!)**
*Determination is the persistence necessary
to fulfill your ambitions.*

—*Author Unknown*

Avoid tempting displays of food and food magazines. Close your eyes and stick your fingers in your ears when food commercials are aired. Skip the all-you-can-eat buffets, stay away from places where the restaurant's kitchen vent is blowing out the mouth-watering smells of juicy steaks. Close your eyes when you walk by a particularly tempting pastry shop (such as Mrs. London's in Saratoga Springs, New York) and try focusing on something else. This might be a good time to start a new hobby! If you are eating dinner at home, serve the food from the stove instead of family style, curbing the temptation to have seconds. You'll think twice about another helping if you have to get up and walk over to the stove. Try chewing gum while cooking so you don't eat a whole portion while "taste testing."

Stay away from people who overeat or who tempt you to overeat. And don't be fooled by the words "fat free"; fat free does not mean calorie free. Fasting is also a poor way to lose weight, because it prepares your body for starving, slows your metabolism, and promotes storage of calories as fat as soon as you start eating again. It's also very weakening to the body. Some people try a juice fast for one day, drinking several glasses of fruit or vegetable juice throughout the day. This is a healthier alternative to simply not eating anything.

Every now and then eat to your heart's content. Reward yourself for a job well done. Eat ice cream with hot fudge sauce and whipped cream, chocolate cake with rich chocolate frosting, a thick juicy steak full of crispy fat, baked potatoes with heaps of butter and sour cream, thick white bread with gobs of butter and cinnamon sugar, chocolate mousse, pancakes with ladles of maple syrup (not all at the same meal, of course!). Enjoy it completely, and then start over tomorrow. Allow yourself no guilt. If you're feeling particularly wretched one day and need food to mend a broken heart, ease loneliness, or banish boredom, just make sure it is healthy food. It's all right to use food as a substitute once in a while as long as the food does not become a permanent replacement for giving yourself comfort, mending your broken heart, easing your loneliness, or banishing your boredom. Call a friend instead!

**Read Those Labels!**
How can we buy food that is good for us? With all the information given to us it is difficult to know what to buy. Reading food labels is the best way we have

of getting what we want and avoiding what we don't want. If the print is too small on the package or there are too many words that sound like chemicals from a science lab, I don't buy it. You don't have to take a course in organic chemistry or memorize encyclopedic data on chemical compounds, just make a mental list of the ones you want to avoid. Saturated fat, partially hydrogenated vegetable oil, and high fructose corn syrup are some "bad" ingredients to avoid. Learn the names of some of the preservatives.

Cooking good food takes a lot of time and effort, and some of us just don't want to be bothered. The challenge then is where to eat and how to make sure the food we are eating is healthy. As a general rule, stay away from fast food, junk food, and convenience food. (Fast food comes from chains like McDonald's and Burger King, junk food includes candy, chips and sweets, and convenience food is boxed and  packaged.) Eat in restaurants that serve fresh, well-cooked selections with several different choices on the menu. Find restaurants that serve alternatives to meat, have some vegetarian items and lots of fresh salads. Salad bars use preservatives to keep the salad fresh, and this may cause allergic reactions in some people.

People who travel, especially those who travel on business, are especially susceptible to bad eating habits. Fast food chains are especially "comforting" when you're in a strange place. After all, that's precisely the point of these places: they're the same wherever you go. That doesn't mean they're healthy, though!

I find one of the best parts of traveling (and I mean traveling on business as well as pleasure) is exploring strange new places—and that includes restaurants, diners, supermarkets, and other "off the beaten path" places. When you are in a strange city, try out the local supermarket. Many of them have prepared sandwiches and small containers of fruit or yogurt. Some even serve hot meals and a variety of fresh cooked food packaged in affordable single size servings. Depending on where you are, you may find that local cuisine is far preferable—in terms of taste as well as healthiness—than chain restaurants. And you can get a good dose of local color, too!

Another travel "hazard" is airplane food—the butt of jokes since airplane food was invented. In terms of taste as well as health, ask for the diabetic diet or low-fat servings. Even the kosher meal is often better than the regular meal.

## Look Right, Look Left

The Swallow International Hotel in London is located right across the street from a Sainbury's supermarket. My daughters and I were staying at the hotel and craving a snack, so we decided to investigate London supermarkets. We crossed the street, careful to look right first, as the cars came whizzing by on the opposite side of the street! Many tourists must have met with disaster crossing London streets, because there are actually large, white painted words on the pavement warning pedestrians to "look right" and "look left." After successfully crossing the street we walked up and down the aisles of the store, delighting in the different brands of food. We decided to try some English cheese and packaged sandwiches, and a couple of bottles of citrus fruit juice. Our bus tour the next day was across the bleak, windy Salisbury Plain to visit Stonehenge, and we thought packing a lunch would be fun. Little did we realize how much more fun we were going to have sitting on the grass gazing at the mysterious circle of stones enjoying our English picnic rather than waiting in long lines with our tour group at the visitor's center cafeteria!

## Cooked and Served with Love
*There is no sincerer love than the love of food.*
—George Bernard Shaw

Have you ever noticed how some food tastes better served by a different restaurant or by certain people? After one of my surgeries, a friend brought my daughters and me a home-made dinner. Served on a lovely platter covered with a cloth napkin and still steaming hot, our mouths started watering before we even saw what it was. Lifting the napkin we discovered chicken with a wine sauce, green beans and almonds, and roasted potatoes, with brownies for dessert. It was one of the best dinners we have ever eaten. We couldn't believe how good it tasted. Could it be that it was prepared with love and caring? Does some of that loving energy spill over onto the food as it is being cooked? This was a completely new idea to me until I started studying different diets.

The mood of the person cooking the meal is an important part of the process. If she is unhappy, anxious, or irritated, the food is supposed to take on these qualities. It is advisable not to cook or eat while in this state. It does make a little sense that if we are all energy beings and are happy and loving while we are creating a meal, some of that energy might make it into the food! I have certainly prayed over food many a night when I've had company coming and it just wasn't coming out right, and while I don't think this is the same concept, my company thoroughly enjoyed their food that evening. Cooking is a creative outlet for many people, so perhaps that creative connection to a higher spiritual plane comes through in the food.

When my daughters and I sit down for dinner, we always light the candles, use cloth napkins (unless we are eating spaghetti,) thank the person who did the cooking, the farmers who grew the food, and the Creator for our bounty. One of my favorite times of the day is when we can all check in and connect with each other, share our joys and concerns, and plan our tomorrows. I highly recommend it.

**To Sum Up**
To practice good nutrition you can:

- Read and learn as much as you can about nutrition.
- Stay informed, read the newspaper, and read books.
- Eat a variety of foods you like in moderation.
- Eat fresh, unprocessed food.
- Eat more fruit and vegetables, less red meat.
- Eat organic whenever possible, wash off pesticides if not.
- Cook from scratch as often as possible.
- Avoid processed food.
- Always check with your doctor before undertaking any type of diet.
- Avoid fast food.
- Choose food wisely.
- Stay away from fad diets and promises too good to be true.
- Listen to your body.
- Talk to others knowledgeable about nutrition.
- Explore different ways of managing your hunger, find one that works for you.
- Support and promote your wellness.
- Balance physical, emotional, mental and spiritual parts of yourself.
- Use common sense, instinct, intuition, logic and reasoning when choosing good nutrition.
- Reduce stress, resolve conflicts.
- Avoid detrimental lifestyles: smoking, drinking too much, not getting enough sleep.

- Take small steps when changing food habits.
- Question everything you read and ask for proof of fantastic claims.
- Reward yourself for a job well done, ands stay positive and happy during the changes.
- Remember Grandma Floyd's old fashioned advice: "Eat your greens" and "Anything in moderation!"

---

After reading this chapter,

- Have you reached your ideal weight?
- Do you know what "healthy food" is?
- Have you started eating healthy food?
- Do you read the labels on all the food you buy?
- Do you know what all the ingredients are—or at least how to find out what they are?
- Do you like yourself as you are right now?
- Do you know a healthy way to lose weight?
- Do you want to come over for dinner?

### "The Garden of Good and Evil"

(Or, the never-ending fight between God and the devil.)

In the beginning, God created the heavens and the Earth. And the earth was without form and void, and darkness was upon the face of the deep. And Satan said, "It doesn't get any better than this."

And God said, "Let there be light," and there was light. And God said, "Let the earth bring forth grass, the herb yielding seed, and the fruit tree yielding fruit." And God saw that it was good.

And Satan said, "There goes the neighborhood."

And God created Man in His own image; male and female created he them. And God looked upon Man and Woman and saw that they were lean and fit.

And Satan said, "I know how I can get back in this game."

And God populated the earth with broccoli and cauliflower and spinach, green and yellow vegetables of all kinds, so Man and Woman would live long and healthy lives.

And Satan created McDonald's. And McDonald's brought forth the ninety-nine cent double cheeseburger. And Satan said to Man, "You want fries with that?" And Man said, "Supersize them." And Man gained five pounds.

And God created the healthful yogurt, that Woman might keep her figure that Man found so fair.

And Satan brought forth chocolate. And Woman gained five pounds.

And God said, "Try my crispy fresh salad."

And Satan brought forth Ben and Jerry's. And Woman gained 10 pounds.

And God said, "I have sent thee heart-healthy vegetables and olive oil with which to cook them."

And Satan brought forth chicken-fried steak so big it needed its own platter. And Man gained 10 pounds and his bad cholesterol went through the roof.

And God brought forth running shoes and Man resolved to lose those extra pounds. And Satan brought forth cable TV with remote control so Man would not have to toil to change channels between ESPN and ESPN2. And Man gained another 20 pounds.

And God said, "You're running up the score, Devil." And God brought forth the potato, a vegetable naturally low in fat, and brimming with nutrition.

And Satan peeled off the healthful skin and sliced the starchy center into chips and deep-fat fried them. And he also created sour cream dip. And Man clutched his remote control and ate the potato chips swaddled in cholesterol.

And Satan saw and said, "It is good."

And Man went into cardiac arrest.

And God sighed and created quadruple bypass surgery.

And Satan created HMOs.

*—Author Unknown (Internet Joke)*

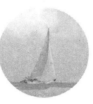

# Full Speed Ahead!
## Adopt Some Form of Exercise

*Mental and spiritual fitness, both dependent on a good brain, are greatly enhanced by optimal physical fitness. Body, mind, and soul are inextricably woven together, and whatever helps or hurts any one of these three sides of the whole man helps or hurts the other two.*

—*Cardiologist Paul Dudley White, M.D.*

Do any of the following apply to you?

- Do you exercise at least three times a week?
- Do you like to exercise?
- Do you exercise with someone?
- Do you have the right gear for your type of exercise?
- Do you warm up before you exercise?
- Do you know which exercises are considered aerobic?

If you answered *no* to more than a few of these questions, you're certainly not alone. Now, this isn't a book on fitness of course, but getting at least *some* regular exercise is important for not only physical but mental well-being.

**Elephant Rock Beach**
*I joined a health club last year, spent about*
*four hundred bucks. Haven't lost a pound.*
*Apparently you have to show up.*

*—Internet Joke*

It is dawn at Elephant Rock Beach in Westport, Massachusetts. Wispy pink clouds stretch across the horizon, clinging to the last bits of night. Dew sparkles on soft green grass and piping plovers dart along the beach searching for some breakfast. A door opens and a sleepy morning riser, carrying a hot cup of coffee, fetches his morning newspaper. Shyly, I wave. He waves back and wishes me well. A gentle breeze lifts a lock of my hair as I bend down to tighten the laces of my roller blades. The road is straight and flat as I glide to the end, carefully turn, and head back. I skate back and forth along the empty road, hearing only the hiss of the waves as they roll back to sea over sand and tiny shells. I finish my sprints and head back to the car. Here I remove my roller blades, grab a towel and my bathing suit, and walk across the street to the beach. I change in the small wooden cabana and walk to the edge of the water, feeling the cool sand under my feet. I tiptoe into the water; it feels chilly but refreshing. I dive in, turning away from the deep water, and swim parallel to the shore. After several laps I begin to shiver and head towards shallow water. Sitting on my beach towel I do some deep breathing for several minutes, and bask in the warmth of the sun and the rhythmic splash of the waves.

Living near the ocean for several years allowed me to exercise in an idyllic setting. Even in the winter I still walked every morning, except if there were a "nor'easter" in the forecast, or ice covered the roads. The ocean kept Westport from getting too hot in summer or too cold in winter. Motivation for maintaining an exercise program was never a problem for me until I moved to upstate New York and experienced "real" winters! It was then that I learned the true meaning of snow and ice storms and discovered that winter weather could be both beautiful and dangerous. Never in my life had I experienced such bitter cold! One morning I couldn't believe what I was seeing and had to squint my eyes at the thermometer to see if it really read twelve degrees below zero. Unfortunately, I stopped walking every day. Warmer weather coaxed me outside again but winters slowed me down. I had to find something to keep me exercising during those ice cold, bleak, wintery days.

Fortunately for me, my sister came to Saratoga Springs for an extended stay one Christmas. I had been living there for three years and by then had stopped exercising completely in the winter. The cancer had progressed into my bones, and the doctor forbade me from downhill skiing. She even frowned on ice skating and cross-country skiing! My sister asked me to find a pool for her so she could swim laps. There is a YMCA in downtown Saratoga with an Olympic-size swimming pool that offers daily rates, so we swam there a few times during her visit. Swimming in 83-degree water was quite comfortable, and the sauna, which was 180 degrees, thoroughly warmed me up. It might have been 20 degrees outside, but we were warm and toasty inside. I had found my new winter exercise!

### The Exercist

> *My grandmother started walking five miles a day*
> *when she was 60. She's 97 now and we don't know*
> *where the heck she is.*
>
> —*Internet Joke*

Finding the right exercise for you could be just as challenging. Do you have any physical problems that could interfere with exercising? Do you live near a YMCA or a health club? Do you have time in a busy schedule? What types of exercise do you enjoy? Do you prefer to be indoors or outdoors? Do you refuse to put on a bathing suit? Do you prefer winter sports to summer sports? Are you recovering from surgery or major illness and need to start slowly? Are you already in great shape and are just bored with your present exercise program and are looking for something a little different? Are finances a problem? If you haven't started exercising for any of these reasons, I hope I can motivate you to start some kind of exercise program today.

What exactly is exercise? According to Gary Yanker in his book *Exercise Rx*, "Exercise is a concentrated form of physical activity that repeats the same movements over and over again, so that the overall body or an individual body part becomes stronger and more flexible."

More than 2,000 years ago, Hippocrates declared exercise to be the best medicine for keeping the body healthy, and this is still true today. A consistent exercise program helps the body perform more efficiently. All the systems of the body benefit, and tissue growth and regeneration are also stimulated. Blood and fluids flow more easily. In contrast, inactivity causes muscles and bones to grow weaker and the body's infrastructure—the skeleton, muscles, tendons, and the skin covering it—literally begin to sag under the pull of gravity. How often have we heard the complaint, "Oh, my aching back?" Older people moan about chronic aches and pains. My sister and I realized we were "getting up there" in age, when we both groaned as we got up from our seats. Laughing, we looked at each other and she asked, "Is this what it means to turn 50?" We both knew it was time to begin anew our New Year's resolutions and start exercising again.

Over-the-counter remedies relieve the symptoms but not the underlying cause of chronic aches and pains. Researchers and health care practitioners all agree that increasing the amount of exercise and physical activity will help alleviate many of the mild aches and pains felt by older people and give positive health benefits for most people of any age. Regular, safe exercise is one of the most important ways to prevent disease and injury. Aging, obesity, high blood pressure, arthritis, diabetes, and osteoporosis are all positively affected by exercising, and there is a positive, indirect effect on other diseases. I used to joke with my oncologist that, except for this little problem of cancer, I was healthy as a horse! Because I have always exercised regularly, my body was in excellent condition when I was diagnosed, so could withstand the rigorous treatments required for me to survive late stage cancer.

Depression has also responded positively to exercise. It has been estimated that between 12 and 18 million Americans suffer from depression, and a good many of those are being treated with Prozac or Zoloft. Many doctors never ask their patients if they are exercising regularly, or incorporate an exercise program in the treatment of depression. According to researchers at Duke University Medical Center in an article in the *Saratogian* (Saratoga Springs' daily newspaper), "thirty minutes of brisk exercise at least three times a week was effective for patients with major depression."

There are a few theories as to why exercise helps depression. Endorphins, opiate-like substances released during exercise, could be one factor. Blood flow to the brain is increased during exercise. Could it be the supportive atmosphere of a group setting that might be missing in the patient's life? Perhaps self-esteem is boosted when the patient completes a self-initiated exercise program and masters an exercise. Whatever the reason, if you are feeling depressed, try exercising!

(Of course, long-term, clinical depression is a serious illness and if the depressed feeling lasts longer than a few days or is more severe than just simply "the blues," please seek proper medical help.)

The effects of an exercise can often be felt immediately, but sometimes it could be days, weeks, or even months before a change is noticed. It all depends on how fit you are right now, what you are trying to accomplish with your exercise program, and how faithfully you follow it. An exercise program should be specifically for you. Your gender, age, fitness level, activity preference, your family health history, your own medical history, and any physical weakness or handicap should all be taken into consideration when designing and undertaking any type of exercise.

Before beginning any exercise program, be sure to check with your doctor. If you are over 35 or have not exercised consistently for the past three months, schedule a physical exam. If you experience any pain or discomfort during your exercise routine, discontinue the exercise and check with your doctor or health care practitioner to eliminate the possibility of injury. If you are under major stress, already have an injury, are fatigued, or have an acute illness, do not exercise or begin any exercise program until the situation has been resolved. During exercise, if you feel any abnormal joint or muscle pain, chest pain, lightheadedness, dizziness, excessive fatigue, nausea, heart palpitations, joint swelling, excessive shortness of breath, or severe pain of any kind, stop exercising immediately and check with your doctor. If you feel fever, tingling or numbness in an arm or leg, severe joint swelling, red, painful or hot joints, or joint immobility, stop exercising and call your doctor. Use caution when trying an exercise for the first time, and go at your own pace. Above all, use common sense when beginning a new exercise program, be realistic about your present abilities, and go slowly.

## Stress and Our Bodies

Exercise also helps alleviate stress. Stress has become our new cultural disease. Stress has been defined as "a mentally or emotionally disruptive or disquieting influence." In our fast-paced "24/7" society, we experience myriad emotionally disruptive influences. Not all stress is bad, we all need some kind of stimulation to remain excited and enthusiastic about life, but chronic, relentless stress threatens our health. When we are exposed to stress, our bodies react to a perceived threat and readies for action. Heart rate increases, muscles tense up, blood sugar rises, breathing becomes rapid and shallow, and circulation to the skin as well as to the digestive system slows. Symptoms of stress include muscle tension, headaches, fatigue, irritability, feeling rushed, anxiousness, and sleeplessness.

According to Dr. Andrew Weil, "Stress raises serum cholesterol and blood pressure and renders the arteries more susceptible to spasms that can initiate heart and brain attacks." When people are stressed, their bodies do not synthesize protein as well as when they are unstressed, so tissues are not repaired or built as efficiently. That is why, even if we are eating well and exercising regularly we can still get sick if we are experiencing great amounts of stress. If you haven't started to reduce your stress levels already, start now.

How can exercise relieve symptoms of stress? Steady rhythmic breathing slows the heart rate over time, stretching eases the muscle soreness, and increased oxygen helps the fatigue. Any low intensity aerobic exercise helps ease the symptoms of stress, and for obvious reasons should be non-competitive! Your problems may not disappear, but your ability to deal with them will strengthen. You will feel calmer overall, so that when you are exposed to stress or personal crisis, it will not have as great an effect on you. Time spent exercising should be non-stressful, in effect cutting down on the amount of time you are being stressed out!

## Benefits of Exercising

What are some of the major benefits of exercise? According to Covert Bailey, fitness guru, in his book *The Ultimate Fit or Fat*, consistent exercise can help the brain, blood, nervous system, muscles, immune system, bones, and heart. For the brain, exercise reduces the number of hours of sleep needed, alleviates depression and anxiety, and induces a natural high with endorphins. For the body in general, exercise decreases the storage of fat and increases the utilization of fat. For the blood, exercise lowers cholesterol, raises HDL cholesterol (the good kind), and helps prevent formation of blood clots. For the nervous system, exercise improves balance and proprioception. Proprioception is our sense of body position—basically, balance and coordination. As we age, we need this proprioception to maintain our balance so we don't fall and break bones. For our muscles, exercise increases fat burning enzymes, grows more capillaries in muscles, and makes muscles more shapely. For the immune system, exercise improves tissue repair and increases resistance to the flu and colds. For the bones, exercise delays or prevents osteoporosis, increases bone density, and makes them stronger. For the heart, exercise lowers resting pulse rates, induces capillary growth in the heart muscle, and lowers blood pressure. (These are all good things.) If you haven't yet been convinced to start exercising, this information should give you some motivation!

Losing weight has always been a reason for people to begin exercising. According to Covert Bailey, "the most efficient exercise to keep you slim is gentle, non-stop exercise that gets you breathing deeply but does not leave you out of breath; that is continuous and uninterrupted, and that uses the big muscles of the thighs and buttocks." Walking, jogging, bicycling and cross-country skiing are examples of exercises for staying slim.

## "I Hate You, Kim!"

If you want to burn fat while you are exercising, you must exercise to the point of breathing deeply but not getting out of breath. Fat can only be burned in the presence of oxygen and when you get out of breath, fat burning stops. Covert Bailey says, "Aerobic exercise stimulates the growth of fat burning enzymes, so you tend to burn more fat even when you're sitting around doing nothing." This is true. When I was younger I could eat just about anything and never gain a pound. Huge ice cream sundaes dripping with hot fudge sauce and gobs of thick, whipped cream. Buttered toast and cinnamon sugar, candy bars, and potato chips smeared with cream cheese. Second helpings of everything at dinner. I was a wiry, active little kid. As soon as dinner was finished I would bolt out the door, jump on my bike and race up and down the street until it got dark. If I wasn't on my bike, I was climbing trees, roller-skating, ice skating, swimming, sliding down snow covered hills, racing a pal, jumping rope or playing touch football with the neighbors. I was the ultimate tomboy, and never stopped for a minute. I was skinny and actually had trouble gaining weight even with all the food I ate. As I grew older and my life slowed down, I still did not gain any weight, as my metabolism was still on high from all the years of constant activity as a child. I could literally sit around doing nothing, eat anything I wanted, and never gain a pound! Yes, I was the envy of those who merely looked at food and gained weight.

## Keep Moving

*The only reason I would take up jogging is*
*so that I could hear heavy breathing again.*

—*Erma Bombeck*

Aerobic exercises burn fat, but which ones are considered aerobic? Aerobic exercises include running, jogging, cross country skiing, mountain biking, race walking, swimming, bicycling, hiking, water aerobics, rowing, walking, jumping rope, and aerobics classes. Machines that are aerobic are the treadmill, aerobic rider, the stair climber, the step/ladder climber, cross country ski machine, stationary bicycle, the rowing machine, and the mini-trampoline. According to Covert Bailey, the following exercises are not technically considered aerobic, but can be adapted so that they give you aerobic benefits: racquetball, squash, downhill skiing, baseball, field/ice hockey, motorcycle riding, tennis, windsurfing, volleyball, dancing, soccer, horseback riding, in-line skating, water skiing, football, ice skating, golf, basketball, and gymnastics.

Golf and other sub-aerobic exercises are still beneficial. They're considered low-intensity exercises, but they still involve some effort. If you are golfing and walk the course you are still getting *some* aerobic workout. Sub-aerobic exercise can still make us healthy and fit, it just takes longer for it to work than aerobic exercise.

Such exercises are not considered aerobic because they are stop and go, not steady and consistent. For exercise to be considered aerobic, we must get our heart rates up to 65-80% of our maximum heart rate and keep it there for a certain amount of time. Most gyms post charts with maximum heart rates according to age, but if you want to find yours without a chart use the following formula:

220 minus your age = your maximum heart rate

Then you can multiply that number by 65 and 80% to get the range of how fast your heart should be beating during aerobic exercise. You must take your pulse at the end of the exercise to find out where you are "in the zone." You can do this by taking your pulse at the wrist for fifteen seconds and multiplying by four to get beats per minute.

Many people do not fit in to the charts. My own resting pulse rate concerns my doctor, but it has always been between 90–100 beats per minute. That is considered to be very fast, but for me it is normal. (Normal resting heart rate is usually between 60–80 beats per minute.) Another way to measure being in the zone is the "talk test." If, for example, you are jogging with a friend, you should be able to talk a little bit without getting completely out of breath, but if you can talk comfortably you should speed up. Passing the "talk test" should put you exactly where you want to be for a good aerobic work out.

How long and how often should you exercise? Much of that answer depends on your age, your present level of fitness, and how in or out of shape you are. The older you are, the more gentle exercises you need, but you need to do them for a longer period of time. You should also vary the type of exercise you do. Try to find several different types of exercises and do them on different days. Remember that resting is just as important as exercising, and a day of rest should always follow a day of exercise with exertion. Your body is unique, and the type of exercise you choose should not only fit your body type, but should be something you enjoy doing. It has been recommended to exercise at least three times a week for a half hour, but this should be an absolute minimum. You could begin with three times a week, and work your way up to five times a week for 45 minutes. A brisk walk could be the exercise to start your day, then practice yoga once a week, and do your intensive workout three times a week. If this sounds like a lot in a busy schedule, look over the things you are doing during the week that are not benefiting your health, and replace them with exercise. You and your body will be a lot happier.

**Dance to the Music**

*I have to exercise in the morning before
my brain figures out what I'm doing.*

—*Internet Joke*

If you haven't exercised in quite a long time, or you have been discouraged by past exercise programs, please give it another try! Following are some ideas to help you get started.

Any type of exercise is better than none. Even if you just get up and dance to some music on the radio, begin today. Get up right now and put some music on and just move to the beat. Do it until you feel a little bit winded, then rest a minute and then continue. There! You've started your exercise program.

Exercise often. It's a good idea to do lots of different types of exercise so you don't get bored doing just one. If you like to country line dance on Friday nights, continue doing that, but you might want to add a 15–20-minute walk three times a week. Getting outside for some fresh air always clears the head. It's a great feeling. Also, exercise doesn't have to be a specific, dedicated activity. If it's possible, walk somewhere instead of driving, or take the stairs instead of the elevator.

Exercise with someone at your own fitness level. There is nothing more discouraging than being left in the dust by an overzealous fitness partner.

Start slowly. If you are out of shape and haven't done any aerobic workouts in a long time, you'll not be running a marathon any time soon. Start with gentle exercise, and work your way up to more demanding workouts.

Exercise for time, not for distance. When your goal is distance, you may speed up the exercise to get there and get it over with. The idea is to keep your heart working "in the zone" over a period of time.

Weather should never be an excuse to avoid exercising, unless the situation is dangerous. There is no such thing as bad weather, it is just how you dress for it. Walking in the rain can be magical, just make sure you wear a good raincoat and all weather shoes. Winter can be just as beautiful, and there is plenty of warm, thermal clothing for outdoor use. Ice can be dangerous, so if it gets icy, use your exercise video. Indoor machines are great if you truly must avoid the bad weather.

Find a sport you enjoy, and do it with others who enjoy it. Bicycling has become a very popular sport, and there are clubs in many areas that encourage riding with others. If you enjoy competition there are plenty of races for skiing, snowboarding, bicycling, dirt bike racing, and just about anything you are interested in. If you can't find a competition, start one! Look for a sponsor and a good cause, and you'll have plenty of enthusiasm and interest.

Do not count calories if you are using exercise to lose weight. The important thing to remember is that your body's metabolism will change, speed up, and it is the increase in your rate of metabolism that will burn the calories and take off the weight. Counting calories could cause you to lose motivation. Don't get discouraged if you don't see results immediately. Nothing beats the feeling six to nine months later when you find your clothes are a lot baggier than they used to be.

Make dietary changes, but don't diet. Dieting has become an obsession in our culture, yet how many diets actually work? Sure, people lose weight, but usually gain it right back once they reach their desired goal. Over time you will lose the weight and keep it off if you continue your exercise program. For now, cut down on fats and animal protein, eat more often, but eat smaller portions. Be careful of "fat-free." This does not mean calorie-free. Actually, one thing that we fail to realize when we are trying to lose weight is that, in some ways, fat is our friend. Fat in foods is what makes us feel full. Fat-free foods don't fill us up as well, and we tend to eat more, ultimately consuming the same amount of—or even more—calories and thus defeating the whole point.

Drink lots of water. Many health professionals insist on eight glasses of water a day, but use your judgment. I found that I couldn't be away from the restroom for more than five minutes at a time drinking eight glasses of water a day, so I cut that down to about four. If the day was exceptionally hot, I drank more water. If I planned to drive for long periods of time, I either drank less water or made sure I knew where all the bathrooms were along the way. Eating lots of fruits and vegetables increases your water intake, and also cuts down on calories.

Use common sense. Listen to your body. (But not if it's saying, "Stop! What are you doing to me? Get me back to the couch and a bag of potato chips!") If you feel pain or discomfort while jogging, for instance, slow down and walk for a while until the pain subsides. You could do a walk/jog until you build up to a full jog.

Take rests between exercise. Your body needs time to repair muscle and tissue from the previous exercise. If you feel especially tired one day, sleep in if it's your day off, or take a nap during your lunch hour. Do not exercise that day. My yoga teacher always ends our yoga sessions with a five-minute "sacred rest." In a nutshell, if you're tired, rest.

It's important to warm up before doing any exercise. Our bodies get more benefits from the exercise if our muscles are warm because they have a larger blood supply and more oxygen than cold muscles, so burn fat faster and more efficiently. The heart is a muscle, too, after all, and also needs warming up. Our muscles become more elastic and stretchable, so we are less likely to injure ourselves. The warm up should be longer if the upcoming exercise is harder on our bodies. For example, if you are going to run in a race, your warm-up should be 15 minutes or more. If you are just going for a jog, a five-minute warm up is sufficient. If you are going for a walk, start out slowly and then speed up.

To warm up, simply do the intended exercise slower and gentler for a few minutes. If you're going for a jog, walk before you jog. If you are going for a run, jog before you run. Pedal slower on your bike. Swim a bit slower. Row slower. Ski slower. Your breathing should begin to speed up, but not be as fast as during the actual exercise. If you are going to be using particular muscles for the exercise, warm up those muscles first.

Over-exercising can be just as bad for you as under-exercising. If you exercise too much, you may be more susceptible to colds and flu, your bone density could decrease, and you could experience mood disturbances. Generally, you'll feel tired all the time, and you may sleep poorly. You might feel depressed, get angry easily, and perform poorly. Symptoms of over-exercising are: fatigue and lethargy, impaired performance, elevated blood pressure, higher resting heart rate, slower reaction time, gastrointestinal disturbances including diarrhea, muscle pain, heaviness in legs, apathy, depression, irritability, joint pain, poor coordination, insomnia, loss of appetite and weight loss.

A friend of mine began a very ambitious exercise program. She had heavy upper thighs and wanted to get rid of some cellulite. She completely cut fat out of her diet, exercised to an extreme, and was sicker that year than she had ever been in her life. She looked drawn and pale and lost quite a bit of weight, although not where she wanted to. After a year of illness, she revamped her exercise program, used her common sense, eventually lost the weight and gained back her health.

To avoid over-training or over-exercising, alternate long, gentle exercise with short, hard workouts. Make sure you are eating plenty of fruits and vegetables, and maintain a healthy diet. Take your rest days as seriously as your work out days, and if you are having any other difficulties it may be time to call your doctor.

## Poor Man's Massage

*I don't exercise at all. If God meant us to touch our toes,*
*He would have put them farther up our body.*

—*Internet Joke*

One of the best exercises I have discovered is yoga. For me it's been a sort of panacea, a "cure-all." Yoga is a mind/body exercise that is appropriate for any age and almost any body type. I believe it is one of the best, most adaptable forms of exercise anyone could ever do. Yoga is performed to stretch and tone the body, calm the mind, increase energy, revive flexibility, and regenerate the body. It is a centuries' old Eastern philosophy and art practiced by a wide variety of cultures. Yoga unites the mind, body, and spirit; enhances health; and improves overall quality of life.

I started yoga classes several years ago after learning and practicing all the poses from a book while living in Portugal. Using a book is better than nothing, but you really must have a teacher show you how to do the poses correctly to get the full benefit. There is a spiritual element that is also missing by doing the exercises solely from a book. The first time we chanted "Om" in class I felt a little silly, but after discovering that chanting "Om" balances the body and unites the energy of those in the group, I cheerfully sang out with the rest of the class. At the end of our session we chant "Om" again after meditating, and I find it gives me a sense of peace and relaxation I never got from any book. The collective energy of the class brings us all up to a higher spiritual level.

During my year of chemotherapy treatment I continued to go to yoga class every week. There were some weeks I could barely lift my feet off the floor, but I continued to attend classes. I believe the yoga helped keep my body supple and stretched which made me feel better. The support and love from my teacher and friends helped too!

Yoga is the ultimate "body tune up." The deep breathing techniques combat fatigue, lower blood pressure, and can even ward off asthma attacks. The stretching and strengthening exercises relieve muscle strains, prevent injuries, lubricate joints, and increase endurance. Bones are strengthened, thus preventing osteoporosis. Each stretch has a counter stretch, which lessens the effects of gravity. After a yoga session the body feels rejuvenated. I call yoga the "poor man's massage."

Perhaps the greatest benefits of yoga are those that cannot be measured. Our culture does not cultivate nor place high value on peace of mind, joy, and contentment, yet it is these qualities that are the most valuable when maintaining a healthy body. Inner peace is the ultimate pay off from doing yoga, and

### The Energizer

According to Godfrey Devereux, yoga teacher, practicing yoga for 15 minutes per day will:

- Work every muscle in the body
- Flush and cleanse every blood vessel
- Calm the nerves and relax the mind
- Massage the brain
- Realign bones and improve posture
- Enhance skin quality
- Improve concentration
- Generate energy, thus creating vitality

many times people will ask me, "How do you do it? How do you stay so calm with all that is going on in your life? How can you look so good?" I attribute much of my healing to the practice of doing yoga, lots of deep breathing, and meditation.

Mental chatter fills all of us with "head clutter," and yoga helps clear any negative thoughts or chatter. So many people have asked me where I get my energy, and I believe that as the mental chatter begins to subside, my spirit is no longer hampered by mental exhaustion caused by negative thoughts, anger, or fear; thus freeing my body of the stressful thoughts those feelings can generate. I feel serene, light of heart, and clear-headed. Even when I feel myself slipping back into old thinking patterns, I quickly start some deep breathing, do my "shrink it down and blow it out" technique, (described in chapter five) and can keep myself calm.

During my cancer treatment I needed to have several MRIs—tests which required me to lie in an enclosed chamber for up to 45 minutes. That was extremely difficult for me the first time. Suffering from claustrophobia, I had to take a pill so I could have the test performed. (Now there's a machine for "open MRIs, but it wasn't available at that time.) After practicing yoga, I could do the MRI with no medication. I practiced my breathing techniques followed by meditation and visualization, and no longer have problems with claustrophobia. (As long as I keep my eyes tightly closed and can listen to music!)

Along with your exercise program and perhaps a short walk every day, I would highly recommend finding a yoga class and joining. Practicing yoga in a group setting once a week will make such improvements in your life, you'll wonder how you ever did without it. You can do yoga your entire life, and there are many classes specifically for seniors. The benefits of yoga are such that I suggest you make it a priority in your life.

### What are Your Exercise Goals?

*I am in shape. Round is a shape.*

—*Internet Joke*

Exercising must be a lifelong pursuit if we are to stay healthy. In order to continue exercising and really make the commitment, you need some exercise goals. Following is a list of questions to help you begin to plan your exercise program.

- What exactly are my exercise goals? To lose weight? Stay fit? Run a marathon?
- What shape am I in now? Is my body ready to do this type of exercise?
- What exactly must I do to accomplish my exercise goals in question #1?
- What can I do to stay motivated?
- How can I incorporate my exercise program into my lifestyle?

In order to list your exercise goals, they must be specific. For example, do you want to "get in shape"? What exactly does that mean? Do you want to run the Boston Marathon, or do you want to be able to walk up a hill without getting out of breath? Be specific. Some general goals might be to lose weight (but how many pounds?), improve your appearance, strengthen muscle tone, reduce stress, improve flexibility, prepare for a competition, or improve cardiovascular fitness.

Be honest and realistic about your body. There is nothing shameful about being overweight or out of shape. Try not to fall into the trap that you have to look good to go to the gym or the pool. If you go to a place where everyone looks like Mr. Universe or Miss America and you don't feel comfortable with that, find a different gym or a different exercise. You don't have to be at the same fitness level as everyone else. You are where you are right now and that is okay.

In order to accomplish your goals, you should be able to measure your success. Losing a few pounds is easy to measure. If you want to lose body fat, find a trainer who can measure that for you. Training for a marathon could be measured in how much further you can run each time you train. Make your goal specific, and check your progress.

Now it is time to take action. Join the club. Go to the pool. Walk every day. If you swam two laps of the pool this week, try for three laps next week. Set a date you want to accomplish your goals. Be specific. Choose a month, a day, or a year and stick to it. Just make sure your goals are reasonable.

The key to realistic goal planning is realizing what exercise can and cannot do for you. Many people get discouraged because their expectations of the exercise do not match reality. They become disillusioned because the exercise didn't give them the results they wanted and expected. If you want to lose 30 pounds, an aerobics class once a week for a month will not do it. If you're "big boned," no matter what you do, your bones will always be big. You will never look like the models on the cover of the magazines. Consider yourself lucky. Those models look like some of the unhealthiest individuals I've ever seen.

## The Yellow Jersey

> *I base most of my fashion taste on what doesn't itch.*
> —*Gilda Radner*

Let's imagine we're at the finish line at the Tour de France. Crowds line the roadway, cheering and clapping. In the distance, we see a small figure, pedaling furiously. Closer now, we see it is Lance Armstrong, hunched down, grasping the handlebars, pedaling toward the finish line. The camera zooms in for a close up. Lance is wearing a bright yellow shirt, black bicycle pants, a strangely shaped helmet, colorful socks and state-of-the-art footwear. Logos scream out at us. Nike! Adidas! Champion! Tour de France! Labels advertise Lance's sponsors. Clothing has become chic in the exercise world. No cyclist worth his salt would be caught wearing anything but the "proper" clothing for a workout. What do you wear when you go out for a jog? Do you "suit up" or throw on a pair of cut-offs and grimy socks? Does it really matter?

## Please Pose for the Paparazzi

Clothing has three important roles to play in your exercise program, and one of them is not to advertise for your sponsors, so don't worry about labels. You may, on the other hand, want to make a fashion statement while out there exercising. Remember Princess Diana the first time she was spotted on the slopes of Aspen by the paparazzi? Frumpy, plain, and unfashionable, she shyly avoided the cameras. After that embarrassing moment, she spiffed herself up, and the next time she was photographed at a trendy ski lodge, she looked as if she had just stepped out of a fashion magazine! If dressing up makes you feel better, then by all means, dress up! Get a friend to take some before and after pictures and revel in your new look!

The second role clothing plays is to optimize your body temperature during the exercise. When engaging in outdoor sports in the winter, it's important to wear thermal underwear to keep your body from getting too cold. Some swimmers stay in the water much later in the season by wearing wet suits. (Members of the Polar Bear Club in the Northeast who jump in icy water on New Year's Day would do well to wear wet suits, but many carry a flask of brandy instead.) Most of the time, because strenuous exercise will raise body temperature, you will probably want to lose heat rather than retain it. Loose fitting clothes made from cotton or other materials that allow water vapor to pass freely are the most sensible.

The third role clothing plays in exercising is to protect the body from injury. In sports or other activities where the body is using the full range of joints, it's important that your clothing does not restrict free movement. Be careful that your clothes are not too baggy or loose fitting or they could get caught in moving parts of machines. Helmets should be worn at all times during bicycling and roller blading. Many skiers and snowboarders are even wearing helmets. Protective padding—especially wrist guards—should also be worn while Rollerblading. Inline skates (like Rollerblades) have been tested for falls, and broken wrists are the most common injury if performed without wrist guards. Clothing can protect one from sunburn as well. Use a sunscreen if you are exercising outdoors, and always wear a hat. Remember to use common sense, and you'll avoid potential injuries.

Footwear is important in protecting your feet from potential injury. When you are deciding which footwear to buy, ask yourself what you need the shoes for. Getting the proper footwear is essential to avoiding injury. Sports stores carry hundreds of different types of shoes for every type of activity. Take your time when choosing footwear, and make sure you get a proper fit. There is nothing worse than suffering from blisters while still a couple of miles away from home. If the shoe doesn't fit, don't wear it!

You may also have other problems with your back, knees, or feet. You can get inserts or extra padding for your shoes to alleviate some of these problems. Check with a professional to be fitted for any corrective devices.

### How Can I Stay Motivated?

*Eat nutritiously. Exercise daily. Die anyway.*

—*T-Shirt Slogan*

One of the biggest problems of any exercise program is staying motivated. We all start out with high hopes and lots of energy and enthusiasm, but a few months down the road our new shoes are scuffed, our colorful outfits are sweat stained, and the jogging course is old and stale. We've become bored, tired, and are ready to quit. How can we stay with our program?

It's important to keep it realistic. If we haven't lifted more than a finger in the last 20 years and decide to participate in a five-mile run, it might take a lot longer to get in shape than a couple of weeks on the treadmill. We should also keep the exercise fun. Once it isn't fun anymore, try something different for a while, or maybe ask a friend to join you.

I used to play women's doubles in tennis, and sometimes things got a bit stale. We usually played with the same people every week, at the same time, at the same place. To perk things up, we planned a party for a mixed doubles round robin and invited spouses and male friends. We rented the tennis courts for the evening, brought food and drinks, played some music, and socialized between sets. It was fun having the men there and it gave a whole different perspective to the game. They gave us some great tips that we used the next time we played. We also gave them tips on how to talk and play tennis at the same time without missing a point!

Doing something you enjoy will help keep you motivated. I love swimming in the ocean, but since I can't do that in Saratoga Springs in the winter (or any other time since it is four hours from the ocean), when I swim at the YMCA, I sometimes close my eyes and visualize being in the ocean. Other times I pretend I am a mermaid and can swim underwater without having to come up for air, or that I am in Puerto Rico, snorkeling at my favorite beach. Sometimes I "people watch" at the pool and wonder who they are, what their lives are like, where they go after swimming. It sounds a bit silly, but it keeps swimming laps from getting too dull. Use your imagination to think of ways to keep your exercise fun and exciting.

Many people find that exercising with a friend keeps them motivated. Knowing that you have to meet someone at six o'clock in the morning for a walk is more motivation than if you were going alone. Give yourself a treat every time you finish a month of consistent exercise. Celebrate your successes, your determination, and your discipline. Buy yourself a new outfit, dine in a restaurant you've never tried, or take a mini-vacation if finances permit.

You could also make exercise part of your social life. If your partner enjoys doing the same sport, invite another couple along. Many exercises lend themselves to social outlets. Before I started my second round of chemo treatments, I used to ski with friends and meet new people on bus trips to different mountains in the area.

## Hitting Bottom
*The advantage of exercising every day is that you die healthier.*
—*Internet Joke*

On a skiing trip to Okemo Mountain in Vermont a few years ago, my daughters, some friends of theirs, and I found ourselves at the top of a very steep, very icy trail, filled with huge moguls. Between the moguls was sheer ice. Several skiers stood at the top of the trail looking down, not moving. We did the same. It didn't look good. "Mom, I'm scared," my younger daughter said to me. "So am I," I gulped. Realizing that the only way out of there was down that precarious trail, I gathered my courage and said, "Well, it's every man (or woman) for him- or herself. I'm going down." And down I went—on my bottom. I must've fallen at least eight times trying to get down. Everyone following me had the same problem. When we reached the lodge, we all decided we'd had enough skiing for the day and decided to celebrate having made it down alive with steaming bowls of soup, hot mulled cider, and a bottle of champagne. What could have been a pity party turned into a lot of fun—comparing bruises and telling our own versions of the adventure. Sharing and laughing perked us up and we decided we would come back and do it all over again some other day.

So whatever you can do to make exercise fun and interesting is a great way to stay motivated. If you prefer solitary walking, jogging, or running, you could listen to music or inspirational tapes, even listen to books on tape and get some "reading" done! Whatever will make your exercise time fun and interesting, and works for you, do it. The most important thing is that you are out there getting your heart pumping, legs moving, body stretching, and feeling better and better every day.

Use your imagination, call a friend, ask your coach to give you some extra inspiration and motivation. Remember that exercise cannot help you if you're not doing it. Exercising should be something you do your entire life, so it should be something you enjoy. Even if you are the oldest, slowest person at the gym or on the slopes, keep going and never give up.

## Gore, Killington, and Suicide Six Ski Resorts

*It's names like "Gore," "Killington," and "Suicide Six"*
*that are less than encouraging for beginning skiers.*

—*Richard Romano*

One day while skiing at Gore Mountain in upstate New York, I passed an older man maneuvering very slowly down the mountain. On my second run, I passed him again. He hadn't gone very far. On my third run I realized it might take him all day to get down the mountain, and felt a little superior, knowing that I could ski four runs to his one. My attitude lasted only a few seconds. I thought, "This man is out here on the slopes, he's not home sitting on the couch whining about his aching back and complaining about the state of the world today. Bravo for him! I hope I can do as well when I am his age!" I never judged another skier again. (After falling several times and spraining two fingers, wrenching my knee, and almost breaking my thumb, I thought maybe that guy had the right idea!)

Reaching a certain age in life does not mean you have to become sedentary. You may have more limitations than when you were younger, but growing old or staying young is all in the mind. My yoga teacher is 68 years old and teaches several classes a week. She is limber, youthful, and quite attractive. She has an inner beauty and peacefulness about her that is powerful.

So although you may not be able to ski down the mountain anymore, you can walk every day, stretch, swim, or do yoga. Staying youthful is possible until the day you die at a ripe old age.

Exercise is a powerful antidote to many of the ills our bodies suffer in these times. Stress threatens to strike us all down, but if we take the time to care for our bodies, we will be able to deal with stress and any crisis that comes our way in a much better state of health. If you aren't already doing some kind of exercise consistently I urge you to begin today, right now, to think of how you can start taking better care of your body. There are literally thousands of books, tapes, and videos on every sport or exercise imaginable. There are gyms, health clubs, and YMCAs. There are sports coaches, personal trainers, clubs and friends ready, willing, and able to help you get into better shape, better health, and better condition. Start exercising. It may just save your life and be the elixir for your soul.

How to adopt some form of exercise:

- Decide what type of exercise you want to do.

- Form a plan.

- Be realistic when setting goals .

- Check with your doctor, describe your plan.
- Discuss with your doctor any limitations, physical disabilities, any problems or areas of caution.
- Make exercising a priority in your schedule.
- Make it fun and interesting.
- Reduce your stress level.
- Practice yoga.
- Write down the benefits of exercise, post it in a prominent location.
- Calculate your heart rate in "the zone" for aerobic workouts.
- Exercise at least three times a week for a half hour. This should be an absolute minimum.
- Bad weather is no excuse for not exercising.
- Make dietary changes, do not diet, do not count calories.
- Use common sense. Listen to your body.
- Make a day for rest.
- Warm up before any exercise.
- Be creative. Think of ways to stay motivated.
- Dress up if that is fun for you.
- Wear protective gear, appropriate clothing and footwear.
- Celebrate your successes.
- Exercise for the rest of your life.

---

After reading this chapter,
- Have you started exercising at least three times a week?
- Have you found an exercise that you like?
- Have you found someone to exercise with?
- Do you have the right gear for your type of exercise?
- Have you started warming up before you exercise?
- Do you know all the aerobic exercises?

# Spiritually Adrift at Sea
## Cultivate Your Spirituality

*In the depth of winter, I finally learned there was in me an invincible summer.*
*—Albert Camus*

Think about the following questions:
- Are you hardened and cynical to the beauty of life?
- Is there a void in your life, and do you try to fill that void with material goods?
- Do those material goods satisfy that void?
- Are you connected with your soul?
- Do you feed and nourish your soul?
- Do you feel close to God, or distant and fearful, even guilty?

We're living in a society that really doesn't put a great deal of value on spirituality. It seems to me that some people use religion as a way to convince others to adopt their beliefs, rules, and regulations. If they don't conform, they are considered "odd," or, even worse, are outcast by the church. Spirituality to me represents belief in a Higher Power that I choose to call God, unconditional love for others, and a non-judgmental attitude. So what I mean by spirituality herein doesn't refer to any particular faith. My point is to show you how to connect to something that satisfies the soul and help you find love and forgiveness and peace.

## So, What's the Big Deal?

Imagine you have just discovered you can fly. You are in the air, using your arms to guide you. You can feel the warm air flowing past your cheeks, the warm sun on your back. You feel light as a feather. Looking first left, then right, you see tall, tree covered mountains. Small white puffy clouds hover over them, backed by the bluest sky you've ever seen. To your right is the ocean, blue, sparkling, stretching as far as the eye can see. Brilliant points of light bounce off the gentle waves. You swoop lower to get a better look. White sand glistens, untouched, soft tiny particles covered by the waves lapping up the beach, now pulled gently back into the sea. Birds call to each other, a soft tropical breeze rattles the fronds of the palm trees. You decide to land in this beautiful place. Stepping down, you walk into the warm crystal clear water, deciding to go for a swim. Swimming is easy. The water holds you up. There is nothing in the water that will hurt you. Out here the water is deep and crystal clear, and you can see right down to the bottom. Sunrays filter through the water, casting light and shadows on the shells and sea grass and coral growing in the depths.

Suddenly you realize you are underwater yet you can breathe perfectly. The gentle push and pull of the waves caresses your body and carries you safely through this magical place.

Your eyes open wide, you had no idea how beautiful this incredible world was. Huge mounds of coral—purple, green, and white—hide tiny purple and yellow fish peeking at you as you drift by. Rainbows shimmer on larger fish flicking their tail fins as they search for morsels of food. Tall green grasses wave to and fro. Dappled shadows move across the clean white sand.

Transfixed, you drift along in this magical world, watching, becoming one with the warm salty water, the soft yellow sunbeams pointing downward. Finally you drift back up to the surface, walk up to the beach, and stretch out on the soft warm sand, closing your eyes, savoring all that you have seen. A whole new world, right there all the time. You just didn't know. You just hadn't seen it before, didn't know it was there. You feel as if you are soaring, filled with joy and gratitude for the new world you have discovered....

Or do you crash to earth, feeling an emptiness, a meaninglessness to all this beauty? Do you ask, "So what's the big deal? What do I care about something I can't even see? What's so special about it?"

## Morally Marooned

*It may be that your sole purpose in life is simply to serve as a warning to others.*
*—Internet Joke*

The difference between those who appreciate natural beauty and those who do not is people's connection to their spiritual side, to their soul. Spirit is defined as "the breath of life, hence life itself." When we say, "Mary is in good spirits," we mean her mood, vivacity, enthusiasm, courage. We may see a spirit, "an apparition or ghost," and our spirit has been described as "a disembodied soul; the human soul after departing from the body." Spirit can be a "supernatural being, an angel, fairy, elf, sprite, demon." Distilled liquors have long been known as "spirits." What happens to the "intelligent, immaterial, and immortal part of man" when we die?

Our soul is defined as "The spiritual, rational, and immortal part in man which distinguishes him from brutes; that part of man which enables him to think and reason. The essence, the essential part."

It is this connection to the essential part of ourselves that gives us the "breath of life" that we crave so deeply. When we have this connection we also have a sense of satisfaction and pleasure, and we are able to appreciate life with all its good and bad without cynicism and lack of caring.

There is a sickness in our world today. Violence has become one way to deal with our anger and frustration that permeate homes, schools, workplaces, airlines, and roads. Litigation has become the norm for solving problems where mediation could work better and without the added hostility, anger and aggression. Attending youth sports has become dangerous from overzealous parents. Our children are at risk of being murdered in their schools by their very own classmates.

What in God's name has happened to us? Why are we so angry? Why are we so depressed? Why are we so frustrated? If we were to psychoanalyze our country, we might look at it and say, "You are obsessed with material things. You are not really facing reality. You do not take responsibility for your own problems, and project blame on others. Most importantly, your spiritual and moral life is begging for attention."

Somewhere along the way, many of us have lost our spirituality. It has become politically incorrect to say prayers in school, even to have a moment of silence, to pray before a sports event, at the office, even among friends. We have separated spirituality so much from our lives that it has left a gaping hole in our souls that materialism has tried to fill. We try to fill that hole with entertainment, power, sexual fulfillment, material things. We believe that if we only find the perfect person for a relationship, the most interesting hobby, the politically correct circle of friends, the right self-help group, the ultimate job, the most luxurious car, the most sophisticated place to live, our problems will be solved and we will find our bliss.

Corporate America has capitalized on this yearning for something and claims to have the answer for our craving. "Experience a Lexus, wear a Versace, dine at Chianti Ristorante, travel to Cancun, spend, spend, spend. Eat, drink and be merry and this will solve all that longing and unhappiness." Maybe. For a little while anyway. What happens when our things lose their luster and the shine wears off the glittering baubles? We buy MORE, and BIGGER, and MORE EXPENSIVE hoping that it will fill the aching void in us. It won't. More, bigger, and more expensive will turn to ashes and leave a foul taste in our mouths, and we will be right back where we started. The emptiness, depression, meaninglessness, loss of values, disillusion with life, relationships, and family will come creeping back, and we will look for someone, anyone, to blame this on. So we have anger and frustration. We have road rage, air rage, school shootings, domestic violence, climbing divorce rates.

Since the terrorist attacks on September 11, 2001, there has been a refreshing change in the United States. More people are praying, more people are placing greater value on their families and friends than on material goods. In a recent issue of *Time* magazine, a businessman was quoted as saying that he was quitting his job and no amount of money could bring him back if it meant leaving his wife and children for long periods of time. I sense a healing beginning in our country. Since I prefer to maintain positive beliefs, I do believe that this will be a permanent change and not just a flash-in-the-pan thing. Thank you for doing your part to prove me right!

## Finding the Pearl in the Oyster

*They keep coming up with new things that nobody wants. Clocks that talk and....You know what we really want? To lie down for a second.*
—*Comedian Paul Reiser*

We've been sold a bill of goods. We are experiencing a timid awakening to the emptiness of material goods and are beginning to ask deeper questions. Where is the joy, the satisfaction, the sense of accomplishment of a job well done? Where has the good life gotten us except into debt and filled with displeasure? Material things are not necessarily evil. There is nothing wrong with living the good life or driving a Lexus. The problem comes when we use these material goods to fill a void in our lives that only connection to the spirit can fill. A funny thing happens when we connect with the spiritual: suddenly these things do not seem so important anymore. We find joy in the simple things in life: sitting by a campfire toasting marshmallows; watching geese fly in formation;

listening to waves crash onto a sandy beach, smelling the salt air; hearing the crickets chirping on a hot summer night. We lose that craving for expensive things that we might not be able to afford. What a relief to those who find the way, a lifting of a burden they didn't even know they were carrying.

By connecting with our souls and the spiritual side of life, we can find fulfillment in our work, rewarding relationships, personal power and happiness, better ways to deal with stress, and eliminate many problems that emerged because we were so disconnected from our true selves. How can we connect with our souls when we are so busy attending to our lives? We must pay attention to messages from our deepest sense of self; we must take care of those areas of soul with regularity, devotion, and time of retreat from the world. This time could be a quiet walk, five minutes of sitting in a meditative state, or actually taking time away from home. There is a hunger for spirituality in our world today that is so deep and powerful and hidden that people don't even realize it. This quiet, reflective time can help us find and feed that part of ourselves.

**The Eye of the Storm**
> *We are born naked, wet, and hungry. Then things get worse.*
> —*Internet Joke*

Between 15 and 20 million people in the United States are clinically depressed and many more suffer from a kind of low level "funk" allowing them to function in the world, but in an unhappy, dissatisfied way. The drug Prozac, an anti-depressant, has become the drug of choice and the "cure-all" for "what ails ya." Three of the top 10 selling prescription drugs today are for depression or ulcers. What is this telling us? Perhaps we just want to pop a pill and hope that everything will be all right. The medical establishment is beginning to look at the big picture and ask "What's going on at home?" instead of just urging their patients to fill their prescription for an anti-depressant.

When we connect with our soul, we find self-knowledge and self-acceptance which leads to self-love and connection with the Divine, which is the ultimate objective of spirituality. This does not necessarily mean an end to all problems and suffering. The first of the Four Noble Truths in the Buddhist religion is "Life is suffering." Being able to overcome that suffering is no easy task. It does allow us to "go with the flow" and to help us re-calibrate our world when we are left reeling from a blind punch from an unexpected catastrophe. Living a soulful life does not excuse us from the troubles that life will always bring, but it gives us a way to deal with them without resorting to alcohol, drugs or other compulsive, unhealthy behaviors.

## God, Please Help Me!

*God finds you naked and he leaves you dying.*
*What happens in between is up to you.*
—*singer/songwriter Robyn Hitchcock*

One morning, I awoke with the most incredible pain in my left breast. It was coming from a lump that had been steadily growing for the past year and a half that doctors had assured me was not cancer. Pleading with God to make everything all right, I went back to the doctor and had it checked again. This time the news was accurate, but bad. It was cancer and had spread to 21 lymph nodes, meaning it had probably spread to other parts of my body—not a good prognosis. "How could You let this happen to me?" I asked God. "This is so unfair! Haven't I led a good life, been a good mother, tried to help others in need? Why are you allowing this to happen to me?"

My answer was not what I wanted to hear and came to me intuitively. "What have you ever learned when life was easy? What personal growth occurred when things were going smoothly? Has an easy life ever caused you to pause and take note of the important things in life? Has your soul prospered and learned to love when your life was flowing smoothly? Did you appreciate life and all you have in that life?"

It was a difficult lesson for me. I swallowed hard and prepared for the long siege that I knew lay ahead if I wanted to survive this. The road was not easy; it was my worst nightmare coming true. Doctors, needles, unending tests, surgeries, treatments that made me sick, and nights when I woke up in a cold sweat, terrified, alone, and utterly miserable.

God was right, however, and, in His ultimate wisdom, showed me that I had a strength I never knew I possessed. He showed me how to take care of my soul, how to ask for help, how to feel joy and appreciation and gusto for life that I wouldn't trade for all the tea in China (besides, all that caffeine is bad for the body!). I reconnected with my soul and found a satisfaction and joy unequalled in any worldly pleasure, yet also allowed me to enjoy worldly pleasures in a healthy and soulful way. Believe it or not, having cancer became the greatest gift I had ever received. Some of us need a sledgehammer to wake us up to ourselves and our souls, and I was one of those people. I thank God every day for that sledgehammer, because reclaiming my spirituality has given me such joy and peace and a solid anchor in my life that I can deal with anything that comes my way and come out smiling, including three more recurrences of cancer. It is so important to connect with the spiritual in times of crisis or tragedy so we do not let our fear and anger at the unfairness of it all hide the hidden jewel that lies amidst the ruins. God will show us that precious gift, but it is up to us to be open enough to allow it to shine through the rubble. That is one of the most difficult things we may ever have to do.

## Bad Things Happen So People Can Be Good

September 11, 2001, is a date that Americans will never forget. I certainly don't have to tell you what happened that day: two hijacked commercial airplanes crashed into the World Trade Towers, causing them to buckle and fall from the heat of the fire. Thousands of innocent victims were crushed beneath the rubble. Hijackers crashed another plane into the Pentagon, causing one side of it to collapse. Heroic passengers on board a fourth plane thwarted it from crashing into its unknown target. The pain and sadness from this series of tragic events was almost too great to bear. Yet out of that heart wrenching tragedy, a jewel shone through. New Yorkers, commonly known for ignoring people in trouble, helped each other in countless ways. Restaurants gave out free food, strangers pulled others to safety when the buildings collapsed, crowds cheered the rescue workers. Normally cynical and hard, people wept openly and held out their arms to complete strangers. My sister and I were watching the horrifying events unfold on TV, and she said, "Maybe bad things happen so people can be good." It was worse than a bad thing, and people were better than good. Americans pulled together that day and the days and weeks to follow, comforting each other and beginning to heal the pain and sickness in us that had threatened to eat away at our very core. People went to church. American flags sold out. Candlelight prayer vigils abounded. Churches, normally closed and locked, stayed open for silent prayer. Groups of people gathered together holding candles and singing "America the Beautiful." Patriotism and pride in our country swelled.

Yet fear permeated the atmosphere. Flights were cancelled. Travel plans changed. Hearts were heavy, and a depressing pall settled over our country. The hole in our hearts needed nothing less than the love and caring of other human beings in order for us to begin to heal. We found that prayer and a reconnection to our souls and our spirituality helped us to be better able to deal with this national tragedy.

I received this poem from an Internet friend, and hope it helps you.

I asked God to take away my pain.
God said, "No.
It is not for me to take away,
but for you to give it up."

I asked God to make my handicapped child whole.
God said, "No.
Her spirit was whole, her body was only temporary."

I asked God to grant me patience.
God said, "No.
Patience is a by-product of tribulations; It isn't granted, it is earned."

I asked God to give me happiness.
God said, "No.
I give you blessings. Happiness is up to you.'

I asked God to spare me pain.
God said, "No.
Suffering draws you apart from worldly cares
and brings you closer to me.

I asked God to make my spirit grow.
God said, "No.
You must grow on your own,
but I will prune you to make you fruitful.

I asked for all things that I might enjoy life.
God said, "No.
I will give you life so that you may enjoy all things."

I asked God to help me LOVE others, as much as He loves me.
God said, "Ahhh....
Finally you have the idea."

**Life Preservers**
Besides being able to deal with unexpected, overwhelming tragedy and crisis, cultivating our spirituality can give us a rich and rewarding life. It can provide a loving connection with our families; an ability to become aware and proud of our cultural heritage and be inspired by nature and protect it from destruction; and create a feeling of unity with our country and our world. You don't need cancer to connect with your soul, but you may need a crisis or personal tragedy to slow you down so you can look at your life, maybe rethink your priorities.

How can we begin to work on our souls? By constant daily attention. We must focus on tending the things around us and becoming sensitive to those things and people closest to us. We must work on our homes so that they feel like a haven from the world, slow down our daily schedules so we don't neglect the important things in our lives; take a closer look at the clothes we wear, the food we eat, the way we exercise, the music we listen to, the air we breathe, the places we travel to, the people we come in contact with. These daily decisions will either feed and nourish our souls or upset them.

Taking care of ourselves implies egotistical thinking, but spirit is nothing like ego. Our souls are the essence of who we are, while our egos represent the more willful side of ourselves. Tending our souls allows this willful side to be taken care of and prevented from ruling our behavior. We can tap into a well of inspiration, an infinite source of creativity, ideas, and imagination that allow us to cultivate our true selves without the willful ego getting in the way. The mystery and excitement of soulful inspiration helps us reflect on and take another look at things we thought we already understood. Our minds can sometimes be like traps, holding us back from doing the things we yearn to do. Ideas, fears and prejudices we have learned along the way become Gospel truth. "That's just the way its supposed to be" we think. "Who says?" I say. "That's just the way we've always done things." Why? Connecting with our souls allows us to step back and take a closer look at our lives, reviewing old beliefs and Gospel truths, seeing things more objectively and without the enormous power of our emotions. Being more objective can help us change limiting beliefs and see things in a different light.

Connecting with the spiritual is the key to living happily, peacefully, and with assurance that all is well, even through crises, disasters, and tragedies. By connecting with our spiritual side, we can gain insight and understanding into life's deepest secrets, receive balm for our souls during times of great anguish and despair, and grow in love and patience, gaining a deeper, more profound understanding of the world around us. We can stop straining and striving for what we need and just ask for it, knowing our prayers will be answered.

Many people express their spirituality and belief of a spirit world through organized religion. Singing old, familiar hymns, following along with prayer books and reciting familiar creeds and prayers, and gathering in a house of worship with others of like minds help many feel close to God. Religion has been described as: "A system of rules of conduct and laws of action based upon the recognition of, belief in, and reverence for a superhuman power of supreme authority." Religion looks beyond this life to the act of creation, what happens after we die, and practicing the highest values in this life. Spirituality is a focus on working on the invisible factors in life and transcending the personal, concrete, everyday things we face in our lives. Each of us must find our own way to worship God, practice religion, and find our spirituality. Attending church, temple, mosque, or other places of worship, meditating, practicing yoga, worshipping with nature, traveling to Sacred Places, or studying Sacred Texts are some ways to connect with the Divine. Our souls want us to live life to the fullest, to live creatively, fully, in love with life and ourselves. When we are not connected with our inner being, we suffer and are not truly happy. Our souls need nourishment, they need for us to express our true selves, to reflect who we really are. It is my belief that, if our souls are stifled, we can become physically or mentally ill.

## Fogged In (Finding the Courage to be Yourself)

*If you cannot get rid of the family skeleton, you might as well make it dance.*
*—George Bernard Shaw*

Celebrating rituals and following traditions are important ways to develop our spirituality. These offer powerful experiences that bind families together. Religious observances, weddings, holiday festivities, birthday parties, and lighting candles at the dinner table  represent some of the different traditions and rituals families practice.

Rituals and traditions will vary with each family and that is what makes them unique and special. They are valuable moments when family life is made a priority. Sadly, many rituals and traditions are being lost to our fast paced and hectic lifestyles. We should not lose the very heart and soul of family life that provide such important anchors for our children.

Rituals and traditions help foster a sense of identity and belonging. When we get together for the holidays and share time together we are, in effect, saying, "This is what it means to be a part of our family and we all have something special to give." They provide comfort and security and help during times of transition. They also offer structure, repetition, and consistency and are something a child can count on.

Rituals and traditions help teach values and impart knowledge and cultural and religious heritage. They are actions, not simply words; a combination of believing and living. Through them we can teach our children what is important to us. They teach practical skills and problem solving in a world that is confusing and scary. Generations can connect and family members can help keep alive the memories of those who have died. Elders can pass on ideas and values from one generation to the next, offering a sense of perspective and continuity. Finally, rituals and traditions can create lasting memories and generate a sense of joy to be a member of that family.

In a world that pushes conformity, it can be of great value to be part of a family that offers us a safe haven from the world and a place we can learn to be ourselves.

Poet e. e. cummings said, "To be nobody but yourself in a world which is doing its best night and day to make you everybody else means to fight the hardest battle which any human being can fight; and never stop fighting."

During my 20s, I attended a church that I would describe as conservative. Rules included: no drinking alcohol, no smoking, no drugs, no Hollywood movies. The members of the church didn't swear, dance, play cards, gamble, or think bad thoughts. They prayed for others, attended church faithfully, served on boards, and sent money to missions. Crusty old Grandma Floyd would have called them "do-gooders." (In a negative way of course.) I admired these people and wanted to be like them.(Except for all the rules. I really just wanted to be "good.") Try as I might, I couldn't do it.

I've always had a rebellious streak in me, and perhaps this was why I was finding it so hard to conform. I believe I inherited it from my Hupp ancestors. They came from Germany to the United States in the early part of our history, and settled out West. Perhaps it was the spirit of the Wild West that caused them to gallop through the dusty streets, whoopin' and hollerin', shooting their guns into the air and, finally, get kicked out of town. I am secretly proud of this rebellious streak and knew that I did not want to stifle it anymore. Being a member of that church was doing just that.

I sat outside on my front porch one summer evening and asked God for an audience. Crickets chirped in the tall grass in the yard, and a warm breeze rustled the leaves in the trees. A thousand stars glittered silently in the Milky

Way. As I reveled in God's beautiful creation, I told Him that I couldn't be like those people and I was sorry but I just had to be myself, wild streak and all. Half expecting a bolt of lightening to strike me dead, what I "heard" instead was, "You are loved for who you are, not what others think you should be. Always be yourself no matter what anyone says or does." I realized that sometimes religion isn't always about spirituality, but may be used to hurt those who don't conform. I quit the church and began my own spiritual pilgrimage. I have never tried to be like anyone else again and have found that people respect me more for living an authentic life.

People who honor themselves and their spirituality are happier and live more fulfilled lives. Living an authentic life is the only way to live. The way will not always be easy. There will be others in your life who will want you to stay exactly where you are spiritually, mentally, and physically. Your role as mother, father, wife, husband, helper, or authority figure may feel comfortable to you and others, and changing that role can be quite difficult. Are you happy living this role? If not, you will never be happy. But if it works for you and you are relatively happy, there is no need to change anything. You must find your own way and what works for you. Do not judge yourself harshly for the path you have chosen, as it is the right one for you at this time.

Our souls have infinite wisdom and can guide us on our journeys. We must listen to that wisdom if we want to make choices that are right for us. If we are leading lives that have no time for quiet reflection or meditation, we will never be able to hear the voice of our soul. We can always find answers within ourselves if we are willing to listen. Once body, mind, and spirit begin to connect we will know intuitively what to ask for.

**Let Go of the Past**
*Memories are like mulligatawny soup in a cheap restaurant.*
*It is best not to stir them.*
—*P.G. Wodehouse*

The key to living a truly spiritual life is to allow the spirit of love, God's spirit, to come through you so you can love yourself and others. How can you allow this spirit to fill you with love? By opening your heart to love, and by living in the present moment. Remaining stuck in the past or worrying about the future cuts off the spark of spirit connection. It is of the utmost importance to let go of the past, forgive past "sins" against you, and be grounded in the present. Let go of worries about the future, quiet those inner voices of fear and grief and anger and anxiety and resentment; they are all ways to distract you and keep you from finding peace within. Daily practice of listening to the "tape" running in your head helps train yourself to stop any negative banter. See Chapter Five for my "Shrink it Down and Blow it Out Technique." Use it often. It really is an effective way to keep your mind clear of any negative debris. Replace any "bad" thoughts with positive affirmations, or picture the Dalai Lama smiling and laughing. Use whatever technique you can think of that works for you.

Learning to love yourself requires a certain amount of reflection and appreciation for who you really are. It is also of paramount importance that you look at both the good and not so good parts of yourself and love and accept both parts equally. You also must be able to allow yourself to have some conflict and contradiction in your life. It's okay to change your mind about something that at one time seemed so important.

One of the most difficult parts of loving yourself is to refrain from judging yourself harshly. How often do you do some self-bashing and call yourself all sort of bad names? How much guilt are you carrying around that you may not even be aware of? Loving yourself means forgiving yourself, no matter what you may have done. Finally, you must be willing to accept and keep those "ugly" parts of yourself that you'd like to get rid of. Instead of getting rid of them, see how they are doing you good and contributing to your uniqueness. They may be qualities that others simply love about you.

### Taking the Bungee Jump

> *It is not the mountain we conquer, but ourselves.*
> —*Sir Edmund Hillary*

Creating a sacred space for cultivating your spirituality and daily meditations can be very helpful. Make an altar using a table, windowsill, desk or outdoors on a rock ledge or garden. What would you like to place on your altar? Use your creativity. Ask your soul what it wants. It could be white candles, purple velvet, or lighting incense, adding rocks or crystals, playing soft music, ringing a bell or a wind chime. When you are ready, center yourself by concentrating on your breath. Breath in, breathe out. Sit quietly like this for as long as you feel like you can, and do it as often as you can. It is the consistency of this quiet time that will eventually quiet your mind long enough for your spirit to begin to peek out. Create little retreats from your busy life. These can be an entire week-end or mini retreats such as keeping a box where dreams and thoughts are kept, reading a daily devotional, keeping a gratitude journal, a walk through the woods, keeping the TV turned off and only watching it certain times, using a piece of sacred art to focus on during a meditation, or doing Qi Chung, Tai Chi or yoga every day.

Once you have begun connecting to your spirit on a regular basis, and are more grounded and less rushed, you can begin to ask questions and receive answers. You can receive any kind of guidance you want.

Do you want a physical healing? Resolution of a problem? Better pay? Spend time with your spiritual side, ask lots of questions and learn to trust the answers. Keeping a journal is a great way to record your experiences with Spirit. Write questions in your journal and record answers. Keep track of any miracles or connections with the Divine and go back now and then to see your progress. Creativity abounds when spirit opens up, and journaling can accelerate this process.

If you experience any fear during this time, ask yourself where it is coming from and what you are trying to protect. Moving through the fear will get you beyond the trap that is holding you back. Remember the words of Theodore Roosevelt, "I have often been afraid, but I would not give in to it. I simply acted as though I was not afraid, and presently the fear disappeared." Developing a strong faith in yourself and God is essential to moving through fear, but is not always easy. I call it the great Bungee Jump. Faith is described as "belief that does not rest on logical proof or material evidence." Many times we are asked to take a leap of faith based on nothing more than just that: faith that what we are about to do will turn out all right.

Many years ago I was working at a good job in Rhode Island. It was stable and predictable, but boring and a dead end. I wanted to take a job in Lisbon, Portugal, teaching English as a second language as my (now ex-) husband was studying there, but had no guarantee that the job would be available unless I was living in Lisbon when it came up. The director of the school guaranteed me the job, but that was the stipulation. I agonized over the decision. Should I stay at a dead-end job in a dead-end town, or take the Bungee jump and move to Portugal on the chance that I might get this job? My friends thought I was crazy when I did just that.

A month after I had settled into Lisbon I was offered a full-time position at the American Language Institute at full salary. I was also asked to tutor executives of a Maritime company and the following year I taught English to the Director of the Department of Education of Lisbon. Had I not taken that leap of faith I would have missed out on the opportunity of a lifetime and the excitement and adventure of living in a foreign country. It was an experience

I value greatly. I have learned that when I want something I must take a leap of faith, and it is still as scary now as it was 25 years ago. Taking the Bungee jump still requires overcoming fears and "what ifs," but I have learned that I must take that leap before I get what I want. Playing it safe and making sure everything is in order will hold you back when it's something big. It just doesn't work that way.

## Got God? (Gateways to Finding Peace)

> *When you're an orthodox worrier,*
> *some days are worse than others.*
>
> —*Erma Bombeck*

> *Emily: Bob, death is just a part of life.*
> *Bob: Yeah, the last part.*
>
> —*The Bob Newhart Show*

There are many mysteries in the world of spirit. No one really knows what happens after we die, but there are many theories. Some organized religions teach that good souls go to heaven, bad souls go to hell. Others believe our souls return to earth to learn lessons, and we continue this cycle of birth and death until we reach enlightenment. Psychics say they can communicate with the "other side" and actually talk to spirits.

My wish is for you to realize that death is not something to be feared or hidden in hushed funeral homes or enclosed in spooky graveyards. Death is as natural as life. In fact, it is simply a life that is transformed from one plane to another. Not many years ago, wakes were held in homes with the deceased laid out on the dining room table. Members of the family took care of the washing of the bodies. Death seemed a natural part of living. Modern medicine can literally bring people back from the dead and the medical community has taken the stance, "save the patient's life at all costs!" Sometimes that cost is high and strips the patient of a dignified and timely death. Remember that death is simply a birth, a passing from this earth to the spiritual plane. It's time to remove the aura of fear from death.

Many people who suffer life-threatening illnesses, or have near-death experiences, may come closer to God or the spirit world and lose their fear of dying at the same time. My sister had a near death experience. During the night while she was sleeping, she stopped breathing. She described the experience to me. "I traveled through a tunnel towards a bright light. There were people on both sides of the tunnel, but I didn't recognize any of them. When I got to the end of the tunnel there was a bright light. I sensed that Jesus was there but I didn't actually see him. I felt the most incredible love and realized that was what I had been searching for my whole life. I wanted to stay with that light and love, but the people in the tunnel told me it wasn't my time. I returned to my body and woke up gasping for air realizing I had stopped breathing in my sleep. I was afraid to tell anyone for many years, because I thought people would think I was crazy. Since then I have no fear of dying, what's to fear? There are just no words to describe the absolute feeling of pure love."

## Riding the Crest of the Wave

*No man is alone. There comes a time when each of us must say, "I can't do it alone." Each of us, sooner or later, holds our hands and says to someone, "Help me." When that time comes, all we have left is our trust.*

—*Perry Mason*

I hope I've been able to help you begin to cultivate your spirituality. And I hope you don't get the sense that I'm advocating any faith in particular, just faith in general. So: take a leap of faith. Open your heart. Use your senses, they are the gateway to your soul. Feel the love that is being offered to you. Give some back. Begin to change your tiny part of the world. You'll be amazed at the results. Developing your spirituality is not a project to improve yourself, although that will be the end result, and it is not a way of being released from the pain and troubles of our human existence, although it will get you through them a lot easier. Cultivating our spirituality touches another dimension. We learn to care for our souls from that place and, in turn, our souls begin to honor themselves. We are able to express ourselves authentically and reveal to the world who we really are. Caring for our souls on a spiritual level allows us to live life in a way that fosters depth and allows our souls to flourish.

We're on our way when we feel an attachment to the world and the people around us and start living more from our hearts than our heads. Our pleasure with the ordinary parts of life starts feeling deeper than usual, colors are brighter, our smiles are wider, our feelings are deeper. Compassion replaces fear and distrust of others.

Our souls are intended to be different, not just amongst individuals, but other cultures too. We need our uniqueness, even our quirks. Our friends and family may be surprised at the new person emerging. It may not be the person they always hoped you'd be, but if we can get out of our own way—overcome perceptions of what others think we should be—then our true selves will emerge for us to love and cherish. Our true personalities will shine forth with a love and joy and zest for life that is worth more than anything the material world has to offer. Take the first step of your spiritual journey. You won't be sorry and you'll never look back.

## How to Cultivate Spirituality

- Create a sacred space.
- Slow down, breathe.
- Meditate, get centered.
- Connect with your inner wisdom, spirit guides, guardian angels.
- Reach out to others on a similar path.
- Practice yoga, go to church, temple or a mosque, be with nature.
- Read Sacred books.
- Travel to Sacred Places.
- Use a personal crisis as a way to connect with your spirituality.
- Pray daily.
- Feed yourself soul food.
- Pay attention to small but amazing moments: sunrises or dewdrops on leaves. See the world through new eyes.
- Stay in the present moment
- Live life based in intuition, inner self, wise self.
- Keep a journal.
- Develop faith. Do the bungee jump.
- Go on retreats and mini retreats.
- Visit your mortality and make peace with it.

After reading this chapter, have you begun to make some changes?

- Have you become less hardened and cynical to the beauty of life?
- Do you feel better about your life as it is right now?
- Have you filled the void in your life in a healthier way?
- Have you connected with your soul and know the soulful part of yourself?
- Do you feel better about being able to react to a tragedy or crisis?
- Are you nourishing your soul?
- Are you happier?
- Do you love yourself?
- Do you feel closer to God?
- Do you feel closer to your family?
- Are you allowing the spirit of love into your life?
- Are you living your life well?
- Are you cultivating your spirituality?
- Have you come to grips with your mortality and feel at peace?

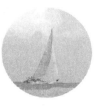

# Living Life on an Even Keel
## Balance All Parts of Your Life

*I began to appreciate time.*
*I don't believe people get enough of it nowadays.*

—*Agatha Christie*

How many of the following apply to you?

- Are all the areas of your life balanced?
- Do you even know how to balance all the parts of your life?
- Do you make good choices in the use of your time?
- Are you flexible?
- Do you know how to prioritize?
- Do you have an organizational plan?
- Or do you live from crisis to crisis without making good use of the "down time"?

If none of them sounded familiar to you, you're probably not alone, but you run the risk of being little more than a house of cards when "the big one" hits. Many people rush from Minor Crisis A to Minor Crisis B and, assuming they ever even have any down time, don't take a step back to stop for a minute and think about how these minor crises can be averted.

**The Ultimate Extreme Living**
*Any idiot can face a crisis—it's this day to day living that wears you out.*
—*Anton Chekhov*

Living in the city was driving the young couple crazy. Traffic, noise, pollution and congestion were causing them stress. "Let's move to the country. We'll love the peace and quiet, the solitude, and the space." The ad for the cabin in the woods was enticing. "Cozy mountain cabin on 20 acres. Miles away from the city, where all you have to do is count the snowflakes." The young couple decided to go for it. "What about all the snow?" a friend asked. "Oh we love to ski, and shoveling will give us plenty of exercise."

The couple moved in. Fall was lovely. The foliage was stunning and they were happy. The first snow came early that year, but they rejoiced in its beauty, the tranquility, and the quiet hush over the mountain. Shoveling was just what they needed for some extra exercise to prepare for the skiing season. Snow came again a few weeks later, and again they cheerfully shoveled and inhaled the fresh, clean air and rejoiced in the sparkle of the snow in the brilliant sunlight. By December, there had been several more snows, each one a bit deeper than the last. The young woman was getting tired. "Could you do the driveway today dear, I'm feeling a bit under the weather." He shoveled the whole thing, even having enough energy to go skiing that day.

January came and so did the real snow. Two blizzards hit, back to back. The snow was too deep to shovel, so the young couple had to hire someone to plow them out. The wood pile was growing smaller, and it was getting colder. During a deep freeze that lasted two weeks, the temperature never reached as high as 20 degrees. An ice storm covered the driveway with a sheet of ice and the four-wheel drive slid into a tree, damaging the front fender. They had to hire a man to sand the driveway.

In February it snowed almost every week, the wood pile was almost gone, and the mailbox had been knocked over by the plow. Feeling isolated, the couple invited friends to visit on weekends for skiing, hot mulled cider, and delicious dinners. When the city dwellers asked the young couple how they were enjoying life in the country, they wanly smiled and murmured, "It's great!"

March came in like a lion with the storm of the century. More than two feet of snow fell, and the young couple was stranded for two days before the snow plow could get them dug out. The firewood was gone, and they were using their electric back-up heat. The cabin seemed to be growing smaller and didn't seem as cozy anymore. Sunglasses helped reduce the constant glare of the sun off the snow. They didn't feel like counting snowflakes any more. "When does spring come around here?" they asked the town folk. The locals just grinned.

By April, gobs of mud filled their driveway and the four-wheel drive sank up to the tire rim in a pothole. The tow truck got stuck in the mire and had to call a bigger one to get it out. The woodman refused to deliver more firewood until the driveway was passable, and the heating bills continued to climb. The nights were still bitter cold. Skiing was out of the question, all their money was going for heating bills, snow plows, sanding trucks, and tow trucks.

A freak snowstorm in April dumped more than of foot of wet, heavy snow on the mountain. A large tree limb fell across the driveway and it took two days before work crews could clear it away. It took another day before the plow showed up, and by then the snow had begun to melt and the driveway had turned into a quagmire. Power was out for four days until the wires could be repaired from the heavy snows that had knocked them down.

In May there was a For Sale sign in front of the cabin.

## The Scales Must Be Equally Balanced

*When you cannot make up your mind which of*
*two evenly balanced courses of action you*
*should take, choose the bolder.*

—*British General W.J. Slim*

Webster's Dictionary describes balance as "a state of equilibrium, to have equal weight on either side." The young city couple mistakenly believed that living in the country would help them balance the difficult parts of their lives, only to find a whole new set of problems. Balancing the different areas of our lives is like juggling. Home, career, family, spirituality, fun, finances, travel, education, and health must all somehow be made to balance with the inevitable problems and crises of life. We don't necessarily have to give equal time to each category, but we must decide what is important to us, give it priority, and then balance everything else. If we are living a somewhat balanced life, when the problems happen, we will be better equipped to deal with them.

It's easy to get out of balance. We must be vigilant to maintain equilibrium in our lives. Have we neglected our health at the expense of our job? Has our career taken the place of relationships? What is the state of our spirituality? What have we given back to our community? Are we happy with our living situation?

Many people believe they have no choice about their circumstances and are stuck where they are. Yes, we were all born into certain life styles and circumstances, adopting ideas and attitudes from our families, schools, and the part of the world where we live. All of these things have certainly shaped our decisions. As an adult, you can look at your choices and ask yourself, Is this where I really want to be right now? Am I truly happy with the relationships in my life? Is my work or career satisfying? Am I in the area of the world that is making a difference in my life and giving it meaning? How is my health, both physical and emotional? How much do I give back to my community? Is my home run well? Are all of these areas of my life balanced?

## The Procrastinators

> *My parents told me I'd never amount to anything because*
> *I procrastinated too much. I told them, "Just you wait."*
> —*Comedian Judy Tenuta*

We all have choices about how we use our time. Do you take the gift of time for granted? We all have 24 hours a day, 168 hours a week, 52 weeks a year. We all share the same number of hours, but how wisely do we use those hours? Why do some people seem to have more time than others? I believe it's because of the way they use the time they have. Look around you. Why are some people doing what they want, living well, happy most of the time, and successful? If you're not one of them—why not? What's keeping you from doing what you really want to do? Is it fear? Is it because you feel like a victim of your circumstances? Are you too busy taking care of other people and not doing what you want to do for yourself? Do you feel guilty when you take care of yourself? Dr. Thomas Arnold Bennet says, "If one cannot arrange that an income of 24 hours a day shall exactly cover all proper items of expenditure, one does muddle one's whole life indefinitely."

Stop right now and write down the five to 10 things that take up most of your time. How you spend your time can show where your priorities are. Is anything missing from your life? If you had only one year to live, would this list change? Are you involved in things that are time thieves? What is the most important thing for you right now? Are you doing it? Remember the words of baseball manager Leo Durocher: "You don't save a pitcher for tomorrow. Tomorrow it may rain."

Emotional clutter in your life could be causing you to "lose" time. This clutter could include people, things, meetings, a job, or situations in your life that are draining you. There are subtle energy drains which steal energy from us that we are probably not even aware of. Look carefully around you and write down some things in your home, your office, your car, or your wardrobe that are either broken, neglected, or need some kind of attention. Have you neglected to get your teeth cleaned, get a physical, paint the closet, change a light bulb, or repair the stove? When you start taking care of the things in your life that are causing mental clutter, your energy levels dramatically increase.

If your life feels a bit chaotic and you are overwhelmed by it all, ask for help. Sit down with a friend or a family member and go over what it is you need changing or fixing in your life. If you are too busy, resign from the boards you happen to be on, stop going to meetings, and turn off the TV. Time spent in meditation each day, even if only for 10 or 15 minutes, will help you slow down, get centered, and stay balanced. Sometimes we continue to do things in a certain way even though it may be damaging to the people around us. We may even be hurting ourselves. You can do a timeline of your life to help you better understand how the past has influenced your present. A timeline breaks down into increments parts of your life that you can dissect and investigate. Draw a line across a sheet of paper. Above the line, mark off each decade of your life, and list any significant life event during that decade. Are any of those life events affecting you right now? It's important to give yourself lots of emotional support while doing this, and congratulate yourself for making it through some very difficult times. Seeing significant milestones or important life events on paper can help you understand why you are doing what you are right now and help you understand what motivates you.

My timeline showed that during my critical growing up years I did not receive enough nurturing from my parents. They had divorced when I was three years old, and my mother, sister, and I moved to my Grandmother's house in Rumford, Rhode Island. My mother had to go to work to support the family when the child support checks stopped, and I didn't see much of her. I really missed her and felt sad and lonely. My father visited once or twice a year. I missed him too.

When I had children of my own, I stayed home with them until they left for college. I did my timeline and discovered why it was important for me to be there for them instead of going out to work. I was giving them the nurturing I never had. In my situation it worked out well for all of us, but in some instances life events could leave us angry or in pain. These feelings could be acted out against someone else in the family and could end up hurting them.

I knew of a musician who seemed angry at the world. He yelled at his wife, hit his children, and was not very happy. His wife insisted he go to counseling and when it came out that he had been physically abused as a child, he realized he was taking out his anger on his family. He was able to confront his feelings and heal the wounds from childhood. He became a calm and loving man.

## Get a Life!

*No one is guaranteed happiness. Life just gives us time and space.*
*It's up to us to fill it with joy and meaning.*
                                                        —*Author Unknown*

Are you ready for a change? Has your life revolved around unfinished business to the detriment of your family? Have you concentrated on a career to the exclusion of all else? You may be ready to head in another direction. If you're feeling like you're sacrificing a part of your life, or are feeling a lack of some kind, your life may be out of balance in that area. Changing your life can be frightening and difficult, but the changes are well worth it. Any positive changes you make will bring you a greater sense of success and peace. If you can bring your life into a balance that is just right for you, everything else will naturally fall into place.

## People Who Need People are the Luckiest People in the World

Relationships are probably the most difficult thing we will have to work on. Human beings are complicated and come with their own agendas, ideas, and beliefs. Many times those ideas and beliefs clash with our own, and we have conflict.  No matter how we try to avoid it, we will always be in relationship with someone. There will be interactions and occasionally strife between men and women, co-workers, family members, children, parents, neighbors, extended family, lovers, friends, acquaintances, long distance relationships, and anyone you come in contact with on a daily basis.

Those who shun relationships may become mentally ill, violent, or commit suicide. We need relationships in our lives to keep us balanced and aware and happy. The people who love us are the most important ones. They shape who we are, add meaning to our lives, and help us when we are in need. Everyone has a need to belong, and having healthy relationships fulfills this need. When a relationship is abusive, draining, or toxic, we need to end it. If you have been physically hurt, emotionally attacked, or constantly feel angry, depressed, nervous, anxious or repressed, it could be a toxic relationship. If you can't sever the relationship, you may need to distance yourself from that person as best

### Taking Stock of Your Life

Ask yourself the following questions to start thinking about your life:

**Career**—What is my ultimate career goal? What is the current state of my career? What would be my ideal job? What would it take to obtain it? Am I willing to take risks?

**Spiritual**—What is my relationship with God? What kind of relationship do I want? If not a god, then what constitutes the spiritual in my life? What beliefs give me solace? Have I given up on spirituality in my life?

**Service, contributions to others**—What contributions can I make to others that will give me joy? How much time am I willing to give to helping others? What have others done for me?

**Fun and adventure**—Am I enjoying life? What would give me the greatest joy and pleasure? Do I allow myself to do this on a regular basis?

**Physical health**—What kind of shape am I in? How is my energy level? What shape would I like to be in? Do I have enough energy to get there? Have I been ignoring any symptoms that may need a physical exam? Have I been "too busy" to pay attention to physical fitness or a proper diet?

**Relationships**—What relationships are the most important to me in my life? Am I doing my best and giving them my all? Am I overlooking anything? Am I ignoring my loved ones to focus on a career? Or vice versa?

**Home**—What is my living situation now? What is my ideal living environment? Am I living there? What would it take to get me there?

**Finances**—What is my financial status? What are my assets, debts, income, and earning potential? How much money would I need to support myself and my intended lifestyle? Do I have a financial plan in place?

**Travel**—Where have I been? Where do I want to go that I have not been to before? Is this an important area in my life?

**Learning**—What are the biggest gaps in my education? If I could continue to learn for the rest of my life, what would I want to know? Do I spend time at the library? Do I have an insatiable thirst for knowledge?

Each one of these areas could take over our lives if we let them. It is up to us to decide how much time we want to devote to each one, and try to balance them all together. It is challenging, yet can be exciting.

you can. At the very least, you should consider some counseling. We often hear of women (and men, too) who stay in abusive relationships out of fear, and it often ends tragically. There is just no reason to stay in a relationship that contains more pain than pleasure.

It is wonderful to have an objective listener when things seem exceptionally difficult. Remember the saying "we can't see the forest for the trees"? Everyone can use some counseling at some point in their lives and one should never feel that there is anything wrong with them when they ask for help.

A psychologist friend of mine helped me several times during my children's growing up years. I would call her in a frenzy asking her advice. She saved my sanity and helped me parent my children in a positive, healthy way. One of the best pieces of advice was, "Don't get in the middle of their fights. Let them work it out themselves." I laid the ground rules (no physical violence or verbal insults) and they had to solve their problem between the two of them. I stayed out of it, did not become the bad guy, and my children learned how to be problem solvers. It has helped them enormously as they have grown, and my daughter tells me that her friends in college come to her for advice.

Relationships in general require a lot of work. Keeping in touch, making phone calls, finding time to meet, sharing dinner or coffee, time to chat, all take time and thought. A friend of mine recently broke her shoulder and was stuck at home. She wanted some company one day, and even though I did have some work I really wanted to finish, I agreed to take her out. She treated me to lunch at Mrs. London's pastry shop in downtown Saratoga Springs, and it was such fun for the both of us. I ultimately managed to finish what I wanted to finish, she was happy to get out of the house, and I got a great treat!

E-mail can be a wonderful way to stay in touch with friends and family, especially if they live far away. My daughter (like a lot of young people these days) stays in touch with her friends by "instant messaging" and she can have three-way conversations with her sister on the phone and another friend online.

But however we maintain them, our relationships support us in difficult times and we need to cultivate them. There is no formula for tending a relationship; it has to be negotiated by each person in loving ways. Each of us has to ask for what we want and need, and we have to learn to listen with an open mind when our partner, friend, or family member explains their needs. It's a little like learning to dance. Sometimes we step on the other's toes, sometimes they step on ours, but if we keep at it long enough, we'll get it right

Healthy relationships should be sustained by mutual enjoyment instead of guilt. "Why haven't you called me?" invokes feelings of guilt. "I'm so glad you called today!" feels much better. Stay in touch with old friends, but always make new ones. Remember the Girl Scout song, "Make new friends, but keep the old. One is silver and the other's gold." A woman once told me I was like "an old shoe" because she felt so comfortable around me. When she saw the quizzical look on my face, she laughed and said it was a compliment. A friend of mine said he likes to have lots of young friends because he is getting to the age when a lot of his friends are dying and he doesn't want to be left alone! It is refreshing and stimulating to have new friends with different interests. It helps keep us young.

## The Good Old Days (Were They Really That Good?)
*To change everything, simply change your attitude.*
—*Author Unknown*

Many of us remember the show *Ozzie and Harriet*. The show depicted the "typical" American family. They never had a fight, dinner was always served on time, and life was good. Daddy never lost his job or hit Mommy, the children were always polite and neatly dressed, and they never had any monetary problems. Sure, they had a crisis now and then, but it was always solved in a timely manner. The show always ended with the problems solved and everyone living happily ever after. Was this really reminiscent of the "good old days?" Did anyone really live this way? As we have become more open and honest as a nation, we have shared our family stories. It seems to me that the "Ozzie and Harriet family" was really the exception rather than the rule. Most of us had some kind of dysfunctional family member or trait. It would be easy to blame the past for our present problems, but this does us no good. It does not help us live a happy, healthy life today. Living in the present and not harping on the past, forgiving past injustices, and not yearning for the "good old days" will keep us from brooding on things we can never change. By letting go of the past, we can have the energy to enjoy the present.

## The Half-Million Dollar Mom
"What do you do?" has come to mean, "What is your line of work, or what do you do for a living?" When people used to ask me that question, I used to answer, "I'm a professional mother." I loved the newspaper article about the Half Million Dollar Mom. A financial planner calculated the market value of the "typical" mother in today's economy. Her jobs included: Chef, nurse, bus driver, waitress, manager, housekeeper, financial manager, caretaker for pets, recreation worker, clerk, nutritionist, social worker, property manager, com-

puter analyst, psychologist, and child care worker. He forgot mechanic, librarian, gym teacher, plumber, electrician, secretary, and systems manager. How do parents balance all of the above and work as well? We should give them all a standing ovation. One mother was criticized because she didn't know that her daughter didn't come home one night. The teenager had been a clerk in a store that had been burglarized and she had been at the police station answering questions. The mother had been asleep, exhausted from trying to juggle all the pieces of her life. I can sympathize with the woman. If we are to take better care of ourselves and our children, something has to change in our culture. Trying to balance our lives in a culture that does not support mothering, and especially single parenting, has become an almost impossible task.

### Building Snow Forts and Fighting Dragons

*I am responsible for my own well-being, my own happiness. The choices and decisions I make regarding my life directly influences the quality of my days.*
*—Kathleen Andrus*

Do you set aside regular time for solitude, silence, and introspection? Do you have a safe, supportive outlet for your emotional well-being? How much time do you allow yourself for fun and adventure? We all need time for introspection, for a little "quiet time." We can get into trouble if we let ourselves get too busy to take stock of things. We could get caught up in the excitement of a job or relationship and neglect all the other parts of our lives. Think of the many things you did as a child. Wasn't most of your free time spent being creative? How much time do you allow yourself every week to do something for pleasure and sheer fun? How often do you use your imagination? Do you only allow yourself two weeks off a year for a planned vacation?

When balancing our lives, we must allow time for fun and adventure, laughter, play, and lightheartedness. We must let go of the cares of the world for a little while each week so that we can face them again on Monday. This is important for our happiness as well as our sanity.

So often, success at a job becomes the focal point of our lives to the exclusion of having fun. We get so serious that we are no longer fun to be around. We believe falsely that having fun is a waste of time if we are to be successful. Many businesses are realizing that their employees actually work better and more creatively if they have regular vacations and time away from work. Having fun allows us to recharge our batteries so we can have the energy, the drive, and the enthusiasm to continue our quest for success.

My daughters' music teacher was working on his career, which included lots of traveling. He was so busy he had to carve out an hour or two from his schedule to come to our house for dinner. Whenever he came to visit, we used to make up funny skits and tape them, or listen to old tapes and make up stories about them. His visits included lots of laughing. After a while, he just wasn't the same anymore. We were worried that our friend was becoming too caught up in his work and not taking enough time for fun. Our next visit proved us wrong, and he was his old self again. He mentioned that he had been getting too busy and overworked, and put a stop to it. He had taken the time to monitor his work schedule, and realized he wasn't taking enough time for himself. He didn't let it go too far, thus avoiding a potential crisis down the road.

Sadly, if we do not balance fun in with our work lives, we may get to the top, but looking around, see what we have lost. It could be friendships, family, or a lover. Our bodies may be tight with tension, stressed and uncomfortable, our friends may have become distant, and we've missed out on a lot of fun! Was it worth it? Are we going to start having fun now? Perhaps. And if you can still continue to have fun at the pinnacle of your career, you have done well at balancing all the parts of your life. All too often this does not happen. Many people have gotten themselves into a rut and do not remember how to let go and have a ball. We may have to give ourselves permission to play or be silly—to be a kid again. Think about your play activities as a child. Pick one that could fit into your life now, and make a promise to yourself that you will do it as soon as it is possible. If you feel any guilt or embarrassment about doing it, feel that feeling, let it go, and have fun! Enjoy yourself! You'll feel burdens and stress melt away. You'll feel younger, lighter, and happier than you have in years. Really let go and get into the spirit of it. Remember what it felt like as a child when you could drop everything and become totally absorbed in what you were doing.

**Pieces of the Puzzle**
Our lives are made up of many different parts. Each one is important and should be cherished, respected, and taken care of. Like pieces of a puzzle, these parts fit together in a pattern that we create through different choices. Some of these pieces may be large, others may be small, some may be fragmented, others forgotten. Yet they all make up the mosaic that is uniquely you.

During our lives these precious pieces may be lost, discarded or stolen from us, without our even being aware of it. We may wake up one day to find that we have lost our balance, become too serious, too irresponsible, or maybe too responsible.

The play *Shirley Valentine*, written by Willy Russell, tells the story about an ordinary middle class housewife and mother who ruminates on her life, her husband, her children, her past. An old school friend sees Shirley, who, at age 42 thinks her life is over, and asks her, "Weren't you Shirley Valentine?" Shirley realizes she no longer is the Shirley Valentine of long ago, a happy teen-ager full of hopes and dreams. She sees through the eyes of her old friend what she has become. Shirley realizes she has put all her hopes and dreams aside for the sake of her husband and family, and she longs to find the real Shirley Valentine, the woman of her youth. She leaves on a vacation for Greece with a friend, and it is there that she finds passion and excitement. When her husband comes looking for her, she invites him to sit on the beach with her and says, "Hello. I used to be the mother. I used to be your wife. But now I'm Shirley Valentine again. Would you like to join me for a drink?"

We must take the time to examine once again all the disjointed pieces of our lives and put them back together in a harmonious way. Each piece has a place in our lives and, because it is a part of us, has always been there. When we balance the pieces of our lives, because of who we are, some of those pieces will be bigger or smaller than others. If we have a job we truly love, we may want to spend more time working than doing household chores. We may need to ask for help or hire someone to do more of the chores we dislike. Don't let other people make you feel guilty about doing or not doing something because they disagree with your choice. Many people I knew in New England thought it scandalous and wasteful to hire someone to clean house. I happen to dislike cleaning house. I would rather be doing something else. Do what you need to do for yourself. Sister Ann Bryan Smollin says, "Let your money work for you. If you hate sewing the hem of your skirt, pay someone else to do it." She's right. Why torture yourself doing something you hate? My own cleaning lady says she hires someone to clean her house! When we balance our lives, we need to do the right thing for us, regardless of what others think or say. This can be difficult when the criticisms come from family and friends, but we can stay strong and do what we need to do for ourselves. I know it makes me very happy when the whole house is clean at one time, even if it only lasts a couple of days. It's cheaper than therapy.

## Are You Sick and Tired of Something?
*Be careful about reading health books. You may die of a misprint.*
—*Mark Twain*

How will we know when we are out of balance? Many times it begins with our health. We may start getting sick more often, we may have an accident, or we may be diagnosed with a degenerative disease and have no risk factors. Our heroine Shirley Valentine's life was out of balance, and she needed to run away with her friend to a Greek island and have an affair to resolve her crisis. If we let the imbalance go too long, it may take a crisis to get our attention.

Have you ever seen a washing machine when it is out of balance? It wiggles and jiggles and moves all over the floor, and if it is seriously out of balance, it stops. It won't begin to work properly again until the clothes are pulled out and the load balanced. When we are seriously out of kilter there are signs before our "machine" completely stops, but we must acknowledge them.

My life had been out of balance for many years, but I had always been taught to ignore difficulties, keep a stiff upper lip, and continue along as if everything were normal. In my family, we were supposed to accept what we were given in life and not ask any questions. Living that way almost killed me! How is your life? Are you keeping a stiff upper lip even though things are not that great? It takes courage to admit things might not be the way we want them, and many times we are taught that it is selfish to want things for ourselves. Many misguided religions teach we should do for others, but neglect to tell us that we must take care of ourselves first. Mother Teresa was considered a saint because she gave up her entire life to help others. I respect her and think highly of her and her accomplishments, but that type of life is not for everybody. I don't believe it makes us less of a saint because we take care of ourselves if this allows us happiness. When we are happy we can actually care for others in a much better state of mind. The caring comes from a place of love, which is infinite, rather than from a sense of duty which will ultimately drain us. However, we need to keep this "self-interest" in balance, too. We certainly don't want to become selfish and self-absorbed and inconsiderate of those around us.

How can we be guided throughout our lives to maintain this balance? It is really up to us—by the choices we make in our lives. If we have gotten out of balance we may hear people say to us "You're working too hard, take a vacation," or "You're doing too much for the kids, take some time for yourself." Listen to these people. Take stock of your life, and decide if what they're saying has merit. Be careful, use your judgment, and make decisions based on what you feel. It is a good idea to talk with a counselor and get an objective view from someone who has no hidden agendas and is not trying to manipulate you for their own gain. Take an honest look at your life, all the pieces: your home, work, relationships, health, and fun, and decide where you might be out of balance.

It can be tricky to balance all the pieces of your life, but it is a skill that can be learned. A friend of mine had $20 which had to last until the end of the week, payday. She needed gas for the car, lunch money for her children, and milk, bread, and eggs. By putting only $8 in the car for gas, and splitting up the rest of the money for lunch and food, she could make it until the end of the week. Unfortunately, she forgot to tell her husband this, and he noticed that the gas tank was getting low, took the $20 and filled the tank. He didn't know they needed groceries and lunch money, but my friend taught her husband the learned skills of not only balancing money for the rest of the week, but communicating with his wife before he spends any more money!

Friends of mine invited me on their sailboat. The wind on the ocean was brisk, and the sailboat tilted over to the side. I was horrified that we would tip over, but my friends assured me we would not. We leaned on the other side of the boat to regain some of the balance, and the boat did not dip so steeply. The keel of the boat kept us from tipping over. The keel is a large piece under the boat that goes deeply into the water, which is the steadying force. When we meditate and stay centered we can use this as our keel to keep us balanced and keep us from tipping over. Regular meditation and inner reflection are the keys to keeping an even keel. We use the term "to keel over," which means to capsize or overturn, and this is what can happen to us emotionally when we lose our life balance. We may find ourselves floundering as if in the water, not knowing what to do. Any type of crisis can cause disruption in our daily routine, and when this happens, it is of utmost importance to get back to a routine as quickly as possible. It is also important to know yourself; to know what you can tolerate and what you can't. Knowing this will save you many heartbreaking moments and possible future calamities—for example, when the big one hits.

A Swahili proverb tells us there are three things that if you don't know, you can't live long in the world:

- What is too much for you;
- What is too little for you;
- What is just right for you.

If you don't know what is just right for you, now is the time to find out!

## Are You Stressed Out?

*I don't do anything without pressure. A physical therapist said, "Get in tune with your body." But if I listened to my body, I'd stay in bed all morning.*

—*Stan Pottinger*

Are you one of those people fueled by adrenalin? Many people believe, mistakenly, that there is little they can do to change the situation they are in. They push themselves to their limits, then wonder why they crash and burn. You know the old expression "burned out"? It is still with us, but now it is called "stressed out." When people ignore warning signs from their bodies, and force themselves to continue working under pressure, they may get depressed, frustrated, and angry.

If we listen to our bodies and they tell us to stay in bed all day, maybe that is what we need to do. Not every day, but maybe once in a while. Do you have to get sick to take a day off from work or school? When my children experienced great stress from our life crises, I would ask them if they needed a "mental health day" from school. That day would consist of sleeping late, going out to breakfast, and maybe going shopping. I'm sure it would have been frowned on by the school, but I believe these days are critical to staying well. When the body is subjected to stress after stress, it never gets a chance to relax. Chronic stress can kill. Try an exercise to see what happens to the muscles when they are constantly flexed. Squeeze your hand for as long as you can. Continue to do this throughout the day. Notice that by the end of the day your hand wants to stay in that squeezed position. Think of your heart muscles squeezing like that all the time as your reaction to stress, and you can understand why so many stressed out people have heart attacks.

Cell phones, e-mail, fax machines, and instant messaging all help us stay in touch but can also keep us in a chronic state of stress. That is OK if you allow yourself time to de-stress, but if you don't balance the time you spend on the computer or working, the chronic stress will take over. The body builds up a sensitivity to stress, never a tolerance. Many deaths are attributed to cancer or heart disease, but how many of those started with stress?

Now we know stress kills, but how can we reduce stress? The vital key to reducing stress is to stop the negative reaction to the stressful situation. We will always have stress in our lives, and even though we can eliminate some of it, we cannot eliminate all of it. But we can change our reaction to it.

Normally when we react to stress, our bodies and muscles tighten, we may clench our jaws, our hearts may beat faster, and we might break out into a sweat. Chronic stress and clenching of our bodies is detrimental to our good health. Reacting to the stressful situation in a calmer, more relaxed manner is the only way to reduce the stresses that we cannot avoid. (Those that we can avoid we obviously should.)

## How to Change Your Reaction to Stress

*People will accept your ideas much more readily if you tell them that Benjamin Franklin said it first.*
—*Words to live by: The Internet*

Several months after I began writing this book my children were in a car accident, and I got the chance to use this method. Luckily I had been using it for the past few months, so I knew what to do when the phone call came. My daughter called me, distraught, saying those words a parent dreads, "Mom, we've been in a car accident." I figured if she was calling me, she was okay. "How is your sister?" They had both been in the car on their way to school. "She's okay. Well, she's not okay, and our car's all smashed." I took it to mean that she might be hurt, but probably not badly. The thought of a smashed car was upsetting, as I didn't have enough money to buy another one. I started to cry, and then thought, "I'm writing a book about this. What would I tell my readers to do in this situation?" I steadied myself, took some deep breaths and drove to the site of the accident as quickly as I could without speeding or getting in an accident myself, continuing to take deep breaths and concentrate on the positive. I checked out both girls and, satisfied that they were basically okay, followed the ambulance taking my older daughter to the hospital for x-rays. The EMTs wanted to check out both girls, so I drove my younger daughter to the hospital. I had an appointment that morning for an injection I needed before my bone scan to monitor the cancer in my bones, and I was 15 minutes late. I left my daughters in the x-ray department and told them I'd be right back, I had to go to the nuclear imaging department to get my injection. I apologized to the technician for being late, but when I explained the situation she was amazed I even showed up at all! I told her I was writing a book on how to change my reaction to stress, and my method worked! X-rays showed my daughters had no broken bones, so the girls went home to nurse minor cuts and bruises. I let out a sigh of relief, and felt a sense of satisfaction with my reaction to the ordeal. (My cancer was stable that time.)

## How Is Your Immune System Working?

*Sometimes you are the bug, sometimes you are the windshield.*
—*Internet joke*

### From Distress to De-Stress

Following is my method for changing your reaction to stress. Benjamin Franklin didn't say this first, as far as I know, but nevertheless the method works and is easy to implement. Read each step carefully. The key to changing your reaction to stress is to practice each step. Be diligent and patient. It takes time to change old habits.

1. **Aware**—We must first be aware of our particular reaction to the stressful situation. What might stress one person might not stress another. You might react differently to the same situation than someone else. For example when my car had problems I used to get upset. I felt tense and out of control. Now I simply call AAA and they either fix it or tow me. How do you react?

2. **Change**—Once we are aware of our reaction to different situations, we can change that reaction. The next time you are in a stressful situation, notice your initial reaction. Become aware of your breathing, and your heartbeat. Take your pulse. Notice if the muscles in your jaw are tight. Check your shoulders and your back. Start to breathe slowly and deeply. Let go of all the muscle tightness, stretch out. Keep doing this for at least half an hour.

3. **Affirmation**—Now start repeating a positive affirmation. I say, "My car is now repaired and running well. I can see it driving smoothly and in excellent running condition. It is paid for and I owe the mechanic nothing." Make up your own affirmation, and continue repeating it. Believe it.

4. **Assess**—The situation, that is. If your car has broken down, do you have a cell phone to call a tow? If not, can you get to a phone? Are you with a friend who can call while you wait in the car? Assess the situation so you can begin working on a solution.

5. **Resolve**—Begin to take steps to resolve the situation. If your car has broken down, call the garage, walk to a phone, or flag down a motorist. Take action.

6. **Believe**—Believe that it's possible to change your reaction to a stressful situation. I guarantee that it can work if you keep trying.

7. **Relax**—You've done it! Congratulate yourself and celebrate!

Life is full of surprises. Sometimes we may feel like the proverbial bug on the windshield, and then there are days we feel as if we could conquer the world. As a good friend of mine said, "Sometimes you're up, and sometimes you're down." In daily living it is hard to know where we will be from day to day. Will we be the bug or the windshield today? Life is stressful. Too much stress can wreak havoc on the immune system as well as on our emotions. The stress response in the body releases hormones that eventually boost blood levels of cortisol, a major stress-coping steroid. Cortisol works to keep the immune system from overreacting and tones down inflammation. As long as the exchange of signals continues in a balanced way, the system works fine.

But if you're already stressed from a divorce or are having a difficult time at work before you get sick, the brain has been sending out a steady stream of hormones that are slowing down the immune system. This makes it more difficult to work at optimal levels, and you will get sick. When my sister sold her house and moved, she was sick for almost the entire winter. Her job causes her stress, so she was already tired, and with the added stress of selling the house and the complications arising from that sale, plus having to move in the winter during cold and snow storms, her body was weakened and she couldn't fight off colds.

Not only does long-term stress leave people more susceptible to infection, it can constrict arteries, weaken bones and muscles, and may accelerate changes in the brain that lead to degenerative diseases like Alzheimer's disease.

Too much stress weakens our defenses, but too little stress can be dangerous too. When someone never has stress, they may not know how to respond when it does happen. If they curl into a ball and go to bed every time there is stress in their lives, they may end up depressed or suicidal.

During our lifetimes we learn how to find balance in the everyday happenings. Most times we probably don't even realize that's what we're doing. If for example one night we don't get enough sleep, we may take a nap the next day and get too much sleep, leaving us feeling groggy and muddled. Too little sleep leaves us tired, and too much sleep makes us feel groggy. When we get just the right amount of sleep, we feel like a million dollars, refreshed, rejuvenated, and ready to take on the world. According to the National Sleep Foundation, American adults average about seven hours of sleep a night during the workweek and seven-and-a-half hours a night on the weekends. About 38% of those surveyed said they take a nap during the weekend lasting about an hour. Experts say the body has a biological need for a certain amount of sleep, and if we don't get enough, we eventually have to catch up.

Some people have physical sleep disorders which could throw them off balance. Some of the more common sleep disorders include delayed sleep phase syndrome, which is an inability to fall asleep at a reasonable time, or get up or out of bed on time. Its causes could be late weekend bed times or odd work schedules. Sleep apnea is a disorder of breathing during sleep. Its symptoms include loud snoring or waking up with a choking sensation. Causes could be attributed to consuming alcohol or being overweight. Often the person has no memory of waking up.

Another sleep disorder is called the restless leg syndrome and is characterized by discomfort in the legs. It can occur while driving, watching television, or during sleep and is relieved by moving the legs. Narcolepsy is the irresistible need to sleep. Symptoms include excessive sleepiness and temporary loss of muscle control. The sleeper jumps right into R.E.M. sleep cycles. Finally, a problem that affects thousands of people every night is insomnia. Symptoms include sleepiness, irritability, and anxiety. A person with insomnia may have difficulty falling asleep, staying asleep, or waking up too early. There are several different types of insomnia, including transient insomnia that lasts for only a night or so, short term insomnia that lasts for about two or three weeks, and chronic insomnia that lasts longer than three weeks. There are over-the-counter remedies for insomnia, but if it becomes chronic, it is important to see your doctor. There may be other underlying causes that could be contributing to the problem.

### Are You Balanced?

*Being on the tightrope is living; everything else is waiting.*
—*Karl Wallenda*

Keeping all the parts of our lives together can be quite challenging, especially if you are not a very organized person. You can bring some order to your busy life, however. Begin by getting a small appointment book to carry with you at all times. I find the most efficient and easiest ones show the entire month and have squares to write appointments. Buy a wall calendar that has spaces large enough to write in appointments, and put it near your telephone. Each day or even each week, whichever works for you, match your appointment book with your calendar. Choose a day or night of the week, and look over the coming week. Note any days that seem especially busy. If I have a busy week coming up, I write each appointment and the time for each day of the week and keep it near my handbag or on the kitchen table to remind me that day will be busy. That way, if I have to cook dinner, I'll know to make it something easy. Figure out a system for you. Sometimes if I forget to take the time on Sunday evening to look over the following week, I'll check my calendar before I go to bed each night. That is not my ideal, but sometimes I just have to "go with the flow."

If my life starts getting too busy and those calendar squares are getting too filled up, I start saying no. I like to leave the weekends free so that I can be spontaneous and feel no pressure. You have control over your life, and you must take control or someone else will. Feeling guilty about saying no is natural, but you have to take care of yourself first. Learn to prioritize. Each January I sit for a while with a cup of steaming tea and think of everything I want to accomplish the following year. I try to limit it to three large items. For example one year I wanted to write a book, plan a graduation party for my daughter, and do chemotherapy. (I didn't really want to do the chemotherapy, but it was not an option.) That was plenty for me to do that year. When people asked me to join a board or help out with a project, I politely but firmly said no. I explained my goals for the year, and if I helped them out I wouldn't be able to accomplish my goals. This takes some discipline, but with a little practice, you can do it.

## Prioritize But Be Flexible

I believe the two most important things to learn in your life if you want to maintain balance are: learn to prioritize and be flexible. One morning while I was writing this book, the telephone rang. I had a thousand different things I had to do that day, and I almost didn't answer the phone. It was my daughter, and she had locked herself out of her car. She was close-by, so I told her I'd be right there with an extra set of keys. The entire ordeal lasted less than a half hour, and while I was driving home I calculated the rest of the errands I had and the time available. I did one of them on the way home, and decided the others would just have to wait until tomorrow. I remembered the line by Betty Jones from the show *Barnaby Jones* when she says, "That's why they made tomorrow, so we don't have to do everything today."

## How to Balance Your Life

- Choose to balance your life.
- Become aware of all the parts of your life that may have been lost, stolen, or discarded.

### Strike While the Irony's Hot

I received this letter from an Internet friend, and I'd like to share it with you.

"The paradox of our time in history is that we have taller buildings, but shorter tempers; wider freeways, but narrower viewpoints; we spend more, but have less; we buy more, but enjoy it less.

"We have bigger houses and smaller families; more conveniences, but less time; we have more degrees, but less sense; more knowledge, but less judgment; more experts, but less solutions; more medicine, but less wellness.

"We have multiplied our possessions, but reduced our values. We talk too much, love too seldom, and hate too often. We've learned how to make a living, but not a life; we've added years to life, not life to years.

"We've been all the way to the moon and back, but have trouble crossing the street to meet the new neighbor.

"We've conquered outer space, but not inner space; we've cleaned up the air, but polluted the soul; we've split the atom, but not our prejudice. We have higher incomes, but lower morals; we've become long on quantity, but short on quality.

"These are the times of tall men, and short character; steep profits, and shallow relationships. These are the times of world peace, but domestic warfare; more leisure, but less fun; more kinds of food, but less nutrition.

"These are the times of two incomes, but more divorce; of fancier houses, but broken homes. It is a time when there is much in the show window and nothing in the stockroom; a time when technology can bring this letter to you and a time when you can choose to make a difference in this world, or do nothing."

- Bring all parts of your life back together.
- Clear mental clutter from your life.
- Do a timeline of your life.
- Choose how you will spend your time.
- Meditate daily.
- Avoid stress when possible.
- Learn how to handle stress in a healthier way.
- Love yourself.
- Share love with others.
- Prioritize.
- Be flexible.

---

After reading this chapter,
- Have you balanced all areas of your life?
- Have you started making good choices in the use of your time?
- Have you started to be more flexible?
- Have you learned how to prioritize?
- Have you started your organizational plan?
- Do you know how to balance all parts of your life?

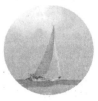

# Clear Sailing
## Choose Positive Beliefs and Attitudes

*Just remember, things are always darkest
just before they go pitch-black.*
—Kelly Robinson, from the show, "I Spy"

Answer honestly the following:

- Do you choose to be happy?
- Can you keep a positive attitude in the face of adversity?
- Do you even think it's possible to keep a positive attitude in the face of adversity?
- Do you find it easy to change?
- Can you forgive others easily?

In today's culture, cynicism is cool. In other words, it's popular to be pessimistic, sarcastic, sardonic, ironic, and all sorts of other "ic-y" words. Anyone with a positive outlook, or the tendency to "always look on the bright side of life" is looked down on as some sort of overbearing "pollyanna" type. But despite the "hipness" of a cynical outlook, is such a worldview really your best friend when a major crisis hits?

It's perfectly possible to be optimistic and positive without being, as they say, so sweet as to rot everyone's teeth

### Colonel Sanders' Lookalike

At one time in my father's life he looked just like Colonel Sanders, founder of Kentucky Fried Chicken. He was living in Florida, and while attending a business meeting in Georgia, he decided to have dinner at a local restaurant. He was savoring the catfish when he noticed people staring at him. Someone sent him a bottle of wine. Another diner bought him a drink—his favorite, Southern Comfort on the rocks. He was wondering what all the fuss was about when a young boy came over to his table and asked for his autograph. It was then he realized that everyone thought he was Colonel Sanders. "What did you do?" I asked him. "Well, I didn't want to lie, but I didn't want to disappoint everybody so I signed it "The Colonel!"

My father made a choice at that restaurant in Georgia, and went along with the assumption that he was a celebrity. Was he wrong? I don't think so. It hurt no one, made everybody happy, and left my father with a funny story to tell. Chances are no one will ever know that it really wasn't Colonel Sanders, and the people who got the autograph will have an exciting story to tell their families. (If any of you reading this were in that restaurant that day, I'm sorry to spoil the fun!)

### Maybe Not So Good, Maybe Good

> *An optimist is the human personification of spring.*
> —*Susan J. Bissonette*

We make choices every day about how we will react to a given circumstance. Will we let a chance remark by someone ruin our day? Will we take offense and choose to make a nasty retort? Or can we let minor irritants slide by and ignore them, not letting something relatively unimportant cause us stress or give us a headache? We can choose to be happy or miserable, and we can focus on all the negatives or all the positives. It's entirely up to us. It's how we react to a situation that makes it positive or negative.

I was driving to my doctor's appointment one morning in November when I stopped to let a driver turn in front of me. Suddenly a truck smacked into the back of my Four-Runner, scaring the wits out of me. We both got out to assess the damage, noting that it was only a crushed fender. The man apologized, we exchanged telephone numbers, and we went on our way. I was a bit annoyed, because I was trying to sell my SUV and now had a crushed fender to deal with. Instead of continuing to feel crabby, I thanked God we were both uninjured and decided to let the incident pass without giving it my valuable time and energy. The man had agreed to pay all damages, so besides being inconvenienced by not having my car for one day while it was being repaired, it was not a big deal. (In fact, it occurred to me that maybe someone working in the body shop will see the "For Sale" sign and want to buy it!)

What could have erupted into road rage was settled in a calm, friendly manner. Neither the man nor I wasted valuable energy on what amounted to nothing. We both chose to accept the situation, assess the damage to both vehicles, and move on. Why should people become angry over an accident? Perhaps it is learned behavior, and if so, we can unlearn it. We can choose to stay calm and act in a civilized manner.

There is an Asian parable about a wise old man and his only son. In the village where they lived, everyone was needed to help work in the fields. One day the old man's son broke his leg. It was serious and the boy was not able to work for a long time. All the villagers came to the old man and said, "Oh, this is so bad." The old man responded, "Maybe not so good, maybe good." Some time later the Emperor's soldiers came to the village and took all the young men away to fight for their country. The old man's son was not taken because of his broken leg. His life was saved and he was able to stay and help in the village. The story goes on with several more "Maybe goods and not so goods," but it illustrates the concept that in any situation, there is more than one way of looking at it. Something may at first appear "not so good," yet after some time we can see that it is "maybe good." I call this "maybe not so good" a spiritual flat tire, a situation that at the time may be annoying, cause us anger or grief, but soon we can see that it was a good thing.

Rudolph Giuliani, the mayor of New York City in 2001, decided to run for the Senate. During the campaign, he was diagnosed with prostate cancer, accused of having an affair, and eventually had to withdraw from the race. It appeared his political career was over—and on top of all that, he had to deal with cancer treatments, as well. He dropped out of the political scene, completed his cancer treatments, and quietly continued working as mayor of New York City. His life changed in the fall of 2001, and he was proclaimed a national hero after his handling of the World Trade Center terrorist attacks. Had he been a Senator, he would not have been able to use his leadership abilities to their fullest and best. His popularity soared, and the people of New York City wanted him to run for a third term as their mayor.

## How Many Tomorrows Do You Have?

A friend of mine knew a man who was meeting his partner at the airport in London to catch a business flight. He missed the plane by five minutes; he cursed and ranted and raged at his bad luck. It was later in the day that he heard the horrifying news, the plane had exploded over Lockerbie, Scotland. Unfortunately, his partner had made the flight. Devastated, yet thankful his life had been spared, he vowed to never get upset again over a situation that at the time seems "maybe not so good."

## Pack Your Bags

*There shouldn't be heart attacks.....or cancer, or anything like that.*
*There should just be a certain age where you have to turn your life in—*
*like a library book. You pack a bag. You go—and that's that.*
*—Rose, from the show "The Golden Girls"*

Do you know how many tomorrows you have? Most likely not. Nobody knows how long they have to live. Being diagnosed with cancer caused me to pause and take note that I might not have as many tomorrows as I had thought, but that was good. It caused me to look at my life and redo a lot of things. If you are living a less than perfect life, ask yourself some difficult questions. Why are you living a life that is less than wonderful? Why are you stuck in an unfulfilling job, an unhappy marriage, a dead-end town?

In the play *Our Town* by Thorton Wilder, the stage manager talks about some of the families in a small, sleepy town. "And there's Mrs. Gibbs and Mrs. Webb come down to make breakfast, just as though it were an ordinary day. I don't have to point out to the women in my audience that those ladies they see before them, both of those ladies cooked three meals a day, one of 'em for 20 years, the other for 40, and no summer vacation. They brought two children apiece, washed, cleaned the house—and never a nervous breakdown. It's like what one of those Middle West poets said: 'You've got to love life to have life, and you've got to have life to love life....' It's what they call a vicious circle." The play is a bit depressing because it seems that life must remain dreary and dismal, and there is no way out. There is a graveyard scene that is quite macabre with the "spirits" of the dead townsfolk discussing events as if they were still living in the town.

Even though we are all terminal, life does not have to be dismal and depressing. In the words of Bull on the TV show "Night Court," "Death is just nature's way of telling you, 'Hey, you're not alive anymore.'" The shadow of death can be what leads us to live a full life. Knowing that we will eventually die can help us live in the moment, aware of what we want out of life, and living with the intention to have it.

We all have that date with destiny that will end our life here on this earth. Why, then, would we waste the precious time we have left? Many of us do not realize that we can change our lives and be happy. Maybe we believe that we can't leave our jobs, our spouses, our towns. We feel stuck by the circumstances surrounding our lives. Old beliefs, fears, and attitudes keep us locked in the prisons we have created in our own minds. We may buy into the philosophy of Susanne Pomeroy from *The Gale Storm Show*, "If at first you don't succeed—give the whole thing up; no sense in making a fool of yourself." But we can break out of jail! We can choose new attitudes and beliefs, face our fears, and move forward. We can say, "If at first you don't succeed, try something else!"

It came as a shock to me when I realized we could choose our attitudes and beliefs. I previously hadn't thought much about any of this and responded to a crisis or problem as I had been taught by my family—which was normally to keep quiet about it, go along as if nothing had happened, keeping a good English stiff upper lip, but churn like a volcano inside. Much of my response to anything was negative, a view shared by most of the people in my family and most of my friends. I reached a low point in my life and began a process of change. One of the things I learned along the way was that we can choose to be happy or miserable. Why would anyone choose to be miserable?

I attended a lecture by Sister Anne Bryan Smollin who told the story about a man who loved to be miserable. He complained about everything. If his wife cooked him meat, he wanted fish. If she served potatoes, he wanted rice. The weather was too hot one day, too cold the next. Nothing ever pleased him. One day the man's long-suffering wife decided she was really going to make him happy this time. She cooked him his favorite breakfast. She made two plates of eggs, one scrambled, one fried. "This time it'll work," she thought. When she brought him his food and set the plate down in front of him, he stared for a minute and then yelled, "You scrambled the wrong egg!"

My life changed drastically when I grasped the concept that I could choose to be happy and do what I wanted with my life. It was not always easy and it was difficult for the people around me. As we begin to change, it forces those around us to change. The people closest to you may be comfortable with their present situation and will not welcome any type of disruption. This can cause quite a lot of stress for all those involved, but the results are worth it. When we are living a life that we love, we are happy, and that has a ripple effect on those around us. Happiness, like yawning, is contagious.

## Beliefs Form our Attitudes

*My dear! I really must get a thinner pencil…*
*this one writes all manner of things that I don't intend.*
—Lewis Carroll, *Through the Looking Glass*

Webster's Dictionary describes a belief as "a firm conviction, opinion, or sentiment." An attitude is "a mental position or feeling with regard to a fact or state." Most of our beliefs and attitudes we learn from our families as young children and continue to form as we grow. We change our beliefs and attitudes as life gives us challenges and crises to work through. When we are children we form a belief about something that may no longer serve us as adults, but the belief is buried so deeply we may not realize where it is coming from.

I have had an aversion to keeping a journal or to write any of my innermost thoughts and feelings for years. This came from a belief that if I wrote something intimate about my thoughts or feelings, something awful would happen. After attending workshops at the International Women's Writing Guild at Skidmore College in Saratoga Springs, New York, I discovered why. When I was 12 years old, I wrote a letter to my friend. I told her I liked a certain boy in our class, but she had to promise not to tell anybody. She not only told everybody, she told the boy while I was standing there. She even showed him my letter to confirm it! Horrified, I turned three shades of red and couldn't speak, wanting to melt into the ground. These feelings of embarrassment and vulnerability had carried through to adulthood, and were standing in my way. Occasionally protective feelings still arise when I am writing, but I remind myself these feelings come from old beliefs and no longer are applicable. How many beliefs, fears or attitudes do you have that are formed from similar circumstances?

## Why Bother?

*Life consists of what a man is thinking all day.*
—Ralph Waldo Emerson

Why is it so important to choose positive beliefs and attitudes? First of all, if we choose to be more positive, we will have fewer problems. How? By looking at problems as challenges. Instead of attaching an emotion to the problem, we can use it as an opportunity to use the resources we have at our disposal. Thus our reaction to the problem can be less stressful. We can prepare for some of the problems by anticipating them. For example, anyone who owns a car knows that at some point that car will need repairs. By putting aside some money each month we will be able to pay our bills when the car inevitably breaks down.

Secondly, we need to choose positive beliefs and attitudes because we will be healthier. We all know what stress can do to our bodies. Many physical ailments can be linked to stress, including heart attacks, cancer, aches and pains, anxiety, asthma, back problems, high blood pressure, strokes, colds and flu, dizziness, headaches, indigestion, insomnia, jaw problems, weight gain or loss, ulcers, rashes, and stiff neck, to name a few. We have been told to reduce stress in our lives. Having a positive attitude can reduce stress by helping us to not focus on the stressful situation or let it take over. No matter how difficult the situation, we have the power to choose how we will deal with it. Mark Twain said it best, "Drag your thoughts away from your troubles—by the ears, by the heels, or any other way you can manage. It's the healthiest thing a body can do."

Thirdly, when we choose positive beliefs and attitudes, we will be happier. Things will begin to look better. All that trouble we used to have will have less power over us and we will have fewer problems. The problems that do come up will be easier to handle. We can choose our belief about a crisis; "Who says this is bad? It is just another problem to be solved." We can take the emotion out of the problem and look at it more objectively. And what point is there to remaining negative and cynical?

I often think of the Dalai Lama, known for being happy all of the time. "How can you be happy after all that has happened to you?" people ask him. His reply, "Happiness is a state of mind."

### I Am Happy—Honest!

*I keep the telephone of my mind open to peace, harmony, health, love, and abundance. Then whenever doubts, anxiety, or fear try to call me, they keep getting a busy signal—and soon they'll forget my number.*

—*Edith Armstrong*

While I was writing this book, I was in one of the most difficult times in my life. I had recently moved to upstate New York, bought a house, broken off my engagement, and was parenting two teenagers as a single mother. That January, the town reassessed the value of my property and raised my taxes over a thousand dollars a year. My house was heated with oil, the price of oil skyrocketed and we had a cold winter. My health insurer went bankrupt and I had to find another at a much higher premium. My daughter began the college search and we needed to visit several colleges. My older car needed major repairs. My water heater needed replacing. My cat got sick. And the doctor told me, "Your cancer is back and has metastasized to your bones." I began a course of weekly chemotherapy and monthly blood transfusions, so had to quit my job. I had been dating some, but now I thought: "Who wants to go out with a bald woman with cancer?" I was in a health crisis, monetary crisis, pre-empty nest syndrome, life crisis, and feeling completely overwhelmed.

I was determined to keep a positive attitude, even with things in my life looking so bleak. Every morning I would wake up and do a meditation. I would breathe into my body, bringing the air up and in, pulling happiness and positive feelings into my body. On the out breath I would blow out all the negative, self-defeating thoughts and feelings. I did this every single morning. I also had an intention for the day, such as: "Today I intend to work on my book, make a nice dinner for my children, and be as loving and happy as I can." I made sure I had something to look forward to, even if it meant only going out to a movie. I visualized the chemotherapy killing the cancer, as well as seeing myself healthy, vibrant, and glowing. If I were having a particularly bad time, I would think, "All I have to do is get through today. I will not think about tomorrow or next week." I asked for lots of loving support from my friends and family.

Day after day I did this, and it worked! A friend of mine had gone to Washington DC to see the Dalai Lama when he came to visit the United States, and was amazed at how peaceful and happy he was after all he had been through. Instead of letting myself get depressed, I would picture the Dalai Lama smiling, and think, "If he can be happy, I can be happy." The oncology nurses teased me when I came in for my weekly treatments and said, "You'll never get any sympathy from us because you always look too good!" And I did. It wasn't easy and it wasn't fun. But by continuing to be positive about everything happening in my life, I felt better, looked better, and got better!

**"Woe is Me"**

*Take your life in your own hands, and what happens?*
*A terrible thing—no one to blame!*

—*Erica Jong*

When things are bad, it is easy to slip into a "poor me" state of mind. Our bodies mirror our feelings. We walk around with stooped shoulders, bent head, sighing with abject despondency. We can get sympathy from others and we should; it's all right to feel sad, overwhelmed, angry, anxious, fearful, or depressed. In order to get through these feelings, we must acknowledge them, feel them, and push through them. Sometimes we get stuck in one or more of these feelings, and may need some help to work through them. Is there an old belief behind that extra sadness? Is that anger more intense than the situation warrants? What's really fueling that anxiety? Everyone is entitled to a day or two of feeling sorry for themselves, but eventually it is time to lift ourselves out of the doldrums and get back to work. If your depression lasts for months, however, you may need to see your doctor to rule out clinical depression.

By the way, chronic depression is a medical condition and help should be sought if depression extends beyond the simple "blahs."

## The Pollyanna Syndrome

*Every year of my life I grow more convinced that it is wisest and best
to fix our attention on the beautiful and the good and dwell
as little as possible on the evil and false.*

—Cecil

When we are happy and see things in a positive light, changes start happening for the better.

We may not notice it at first, but over time our entire beings will begin to express that positive stance. The furrow over our brows will disappear, we'll smile more, our eyes will light up, we'll carry our bodies straighter, and there will be more spring in our step. There are two ways to look at things, either positively or negatively. There will always be both in your life and you can either focus on the positive or the negative. If you choose to focus on the positive your life will truly change for the better.

I was having breakfast one morning with my "McDonald's Guys," a group of retired men who meet every morning for coffee and companionship. One morning we were discussing one of the men's daughters. She had been in a car accident several years before, and had suffered crushed hips. Her hips were degenerating, and if she didn't have hip replacement surgery, she would eventually be crippled. Someone said, "Oh isn't that just awful. To have to go through such a difficult surgery at such a young age!" My comment was, "How wonderful! Isn't it great there is such an operation to replace her hips so that she won't be crippled and end up in a wheelchair!" My sister sometimes gets annoyed with me because I turn everything around to find the positive. My Grandmother used to say, "Oh there's Pollyanna talking again." One day my sister said, "Oh, be quiet, Kim. Let me be grumpy today!"

We all know people who thrive on the negative. If you choose to focus on the positive instead of the negative, these people may begin to disappear from your life, or they may begin to look at things differently. (Or they may tell you to be quiet and let them be grumpy!) Getting stress and negativity out of your life and doing what you love to do will not only give you incredible amounts of energy, it will increase your level of health.

What is the "Pollyanna Syndrome?" *Pollyanna* is a classic movie, first released in 1920, then again by Walt Disney in 1960 starring Haley Mills. Pollyanna is an orphan, sent to live with her "crotchety" aunt in a small New England town. The people in the town are as ill-tempered as her aunt. With her indomitable will to see the good side of even the worst situations, Pollyanna transforms the community and teaches the townsfolk the joys and pleasures that can be enjoyed in life.

I call it the Pollyanna Syndrome to be able to see the positive side of everything. This does not mean we should ignore tragedy and sadness or stick our heads in the sand, but accept what God has given us and make the best of it.

## This Is the Last Place I Want to Be

Change usually does not happen overnight. When I was in the middle of my money, health, and life crisis, I felt like I was in the middle of a battlefield, hunkered down with the troops. Bullets were screaming and whizzing over my head. This was the last place on earth I wanted to be. I was scared, tired, and lonely. But the battle was waging and if I stood up and tried to walk away, I would be shot down. The only thing I could do was reach inside to find my courage, fight the battle, and somehow make it out of there alive.

When things get bad and we feel like we are in the midst of battle, we can be overwhelmed by the enormity of the situation. Sometimes the only thing we can do is slow down, take a deep breath, and sit quietly. Breathing is the best way to relax the body. It can put us in a much calmer place. The problems will not go away, but our reaction to them is changed, we can think more clearly and experience less stress. When we have less stress we can be more resourceful dealing with the present situation and ultimately make better decisions.

## Start Making Some Changes

*She changed her mind, but it didn't work
any better than the old one.*

—Henny Youngman

How can we start making changes in our lives? First we have to make an honest assessment of things we are not happy with. Then we have to have a willingness to release old beliefs, thought patterns, and attitudes. Sometimes when we start working on releasing an old pattern, things seem to get worse for awhile. This is not bad and indicates that things are starting to move forward. It is usually an opportunity to look at the old pattern, discover why you believe it, and work through it. When you have setbacks don't give up, keep going, and things will eventually get better.

We can change our way of thinking. We must realize that we control our minds, our minds don't control us. In the past, you may have allowed your mind to think a certain way, but you can train your mind to think any way you want it to.

Your present way of thinking has developed over time from beliefs and attitudes learned as you were growing up, observing different situations and choosing beliefs and attitudes based on circumstances at that time. The only thing you have control over are the thoughts you are thinking right now. The past is past, the future is unknown. The power is in the present moment. You can choose and control your thoughts, it just takes a little discipline. You are not a victim of your life, your thoughts, or your present situation. Remember that you are in control, and you are the master of your own mind.

In the book *21 Mine* by Jeffrey G. Kelly, there is a remedy for the prisoners to follow in order to change their old habits of responding to a negative situation. I found it helpful. You can use it to begin to make changes in your life. Use this formula when you set goals for yourself. It makes them manageable.

*S.M.A.R.T.:*
Specific
Measurable
Attainable
Realistic
Timely

## How To Make Changes in Our Attitudes

1. Become clear on what you want to change in your life.

2. Say to yourself: I have created this situation in my life or allowed it to happen. I am willing to let go of the belief that is responsible for this situation.

3. Ask yourself: Do I really mean this? Do I really want to change this? Am I ready to become unstuck?

4. Look at the past: What ideas, beliefs, or attitudes are causing the present situation?

5. Notice any fears, blocks, or resistance that come up.

6. Face the fears, look at the block or resistance and let it go.

7. Enjoy the new change!

8. Use the S.M.A.R.T. technique to help you make your changes.

**Forgiveness**
*Carrying a grudge is like a run in a stocking—it can only get worse.*
*Forgiveness is the answer.*
—*Author Unknown*

When you begin your new thinking process, your old thinking process is almost sure to rebel. Remember when the no smoking rule took effect in airplanes, restaurants, and hospitals? Complaints abounded. People were enraged. They wrote their representatives and loudly voiced their complaints. Yet now it seems unthinkable for anyone to smoke on an airplane or in a hospital. Be prepared for some complaining from your old thinking patterns, don't give in, and soon it will seem normal. Many times resistance to new thinking comes from old hurts and resentments. We believe that if we hold on to that anger or hurt, we can somehow punish that person who injured us, but in actuality, we are only hurting ourselves. Holding on to hurts and resentments can lead to many health problems, including cancer. By forgiving the people who hurt us, we can release the past, let go of the hurt or anger, move on, and begin to love ourselves. True healing can only happen after we forgive, for it allows love into our hearts. Love is the greatest healer there is.

Forgiveness is one of the hardest things for people to do. Causes of ill will towards others may stem from regret, sadness, hurt, fear, guilt, blame, anger, resentment, or desire for revenge. Forgiving someone does not mean you condone their actions or make them right. What they did was wrong. And forgiving them does not mean you have to be their best friend. It only means you can forgive them and let them go from your life. How freeing! The person you want to hurt probably does not even know or care about your past grievances; it doesn't bother them a bit. Forgive, forget, and let go. What's past is past. You may need to forgive yourself for something. What you did may have been wrong or hurt someone. If you can go to that person and ask for their forgiveness, do it. If not, forgive yourself anyway. Old thought patterns can be changed, and you can learn to forgive even if you have to let God do it for you.

I was having an exceptionally hard time forgiving my Grandmother for physically abusing me as a child. I could not forgive her. So I asked God to forgive her through me, and this worked. Eventually I was able to forgive her myself, and even though she has died, I can sincerely wish her well. What a feeling of relief and peace! It feels as if a huge load has been lifted from my body.

---

### Exercise: Forgiving a Person

1. Find a quiet spot, light a candle and burn some incense.
2. Take a few deep breaths, and sit quietly.
3. Imagine the person you need to forgive.
4. Say the person's name, and then say "I forgive you for _____ _____."
5. Imagine the person saying, "Thank you, you are now set free."
6. Forgive all injustices from this person.
7. Let go of all feelings of resentment, anger, sadness, and revenge after feeling them fully.
8. Forgive yourself, saying, "I forgive myself for _____ _____."
9. Do this at least once a week until you have truly let go and moved on.

**With a Vengeance**
> *Always forgive your enemies; nothing annoys them so much.*
> —*Oscar Wilde*

Sometimes there is a place in us that desires revenge on the people who hurt us. This is normal and should be addressed. One way to release the feelings of revenge is to picture the person you are angry with. Ask yourself what they need to do in order for you to be able to forgive them. Visualize them doing this. Imagine it happening in detail. Ask yourself how long they need to suffer and do penance. When you feel okay about it, let it go, let it be done and over with, forever. This can be freeing, but should only be done once. It is not healthy to hang on to feelings of resentment and revenge. After the terrorist attacks on the United States on September 11, 2001, there was a lot of resentment towards those responsible. People were angry and wanted revenge. That is a normal response to an event such as this. Eventually those same people who wanted revenge must forgive, if only to help themselves move beyond the tragedy.

**What Do You Want to Change?**
When you realize that you can make a difference in your own life, it may be difficult to know where to begin. Start by making a list of the areas you want to start working on. In my case, it was my entire life. Since this was a bit daunting, I had to look at things in my life and ask myself what was happening that was good, what was a priority, and what could be worked on later.

When you begin to make changes in your life, you should look at your areas of strengths as well as areas to be improved. We all have some of each. During one of my blood transfusions a woman was bemoaning the fact that she was going to turn 40 years old on her next birthday. My comment to her was, "Consider the alternative!" That woman needed to change her attitude about growing older. Rose of the "Golden Girls," had the right idea when she said, "My mother always used to say, 'The older you get, the better you get—unless you're a banana!'" Do you have any attitude adjustments to make?

**"Shrink It Down and Blow It Out"**
The next step to changing an attitude or belief is to begin affirming them. If you want more money in your life begin by saying, "I now have more money in my life." Make sure the affirmation is in the present tense. Use of the word "will" indicates some future time so the idea never manifests. Meditate on the belief, open your mind to infinite possibilities, and watch what happens. If

you secretly believe that nothing will happen, then nothing will happen. If you believe it will happen, then it will. Try an exercise to see if this really works. For the next three months begin affirming something you want or need. Take a few minutes to decide what you want to work on, write down the affirmation, and meditate on it every day. Repeat the affirmation several times a day, and believe that you will reach your desired goal. At the end of three months check in and see what progress you have made.

My younger daughter's art class had planned a trip to New York City. It was in February, and she didn't have any winter boots, only sneakers. Her feet were cold and she wanted boots. She has a narrow foot, and it's difficult to find shoes that fit. She kept lamenting that she would never find boots before the trip. I assured her that this was true. I suggested she affirm instead. "I now have the perfect boots in the perfect size and the money to buy them," and see what happened. Being a teenager, she was skeptical, but went along with it because she really wanted the boots. After a few days of this, we went to our favorite shoe store in Saratoga. She tried on the boots she liked, but they did not have them in her size. She gave me an accusing look. The clerk said, "Sorry we don't have them in your size, but we can order them for you from our other store." She got the boots the day before her trip.

I asked for more abundance during my monetary crisis. One day I was driving home from church and stopped at a yard sale. I love earrings, and when I saw a table full of them, I knew I had hit the mother lode. Great long, dangling earrings, just the kind I love. "How much do you want for the earrings?" The man said that his wife wanted 25¢ a pair. He explained that he owned a retail shop and wanted to reduce his inventory. I left with 30 pairs of earrings, and a feeling of absolute astonishment that this way of thinking really worked!

I agree with the great philosopher Cecil when he said to fix our attention on the beautiful and dwell as little as possible on the evil and false (or the negative). It's a great idea, but extremely difficult to actually do. With all the negative thoughts churning in our heads, how can we possibly dwell only on the good? I have a system I use that I call the "Shrink it down and blow it out" technique. I use it often.

When a negative person, thought, or image comes into your mind, visualize shrinking them to a tiny size. Remember the movie, *Honey I Shrunk the Kids*? The main character had invented a "shrinking machine" and had accidentally shrunk his children. They were so small that blades of grass seemed as tall as giant sequoias. Create a "shrinking machine" in your mind, and shrink the negative person, image, or thought. Then visually place them at the top of your nasal cavity. Take in a breath of air and blow out, seeing that tiny person, image, or thought blowing out of your nose. It's especially gratifying to imagine negative people being tossed about as they are flying through the air.

## Change Is a Process and Takes Time
*It is hard to fight an enemy who has outposts in your head.*
—*Sally Kempton*

Remember that change is a process. It takes time. We all come with ideas and beliefs that we have fostered for many years, and these beliefs grab hold of us and do not want to let us go. Feelings of guilt may arise if your new ideas go against old family beliefs. Wherever there is change, there may be fear. Fear and change normally go hand in hand. Fear is an uncomfortable feeling, but that is all it is—a feeling. Respect your fear, thank it for trying to protect you, but if the situation is not a dangerous one and it is ultimately for your good, push through your fear. If you face your fear, you can transform it into courage. Take control of the fear by acknowledging it, admitting that you have the fear, feeling it fully, and then moving forward with the activity that induced it. If you run from fear, especially if it is from an unknown, it can start growing and can keep you from experiencing a full life. Give yourself a pat on the back for even attempting the fearful activity. Remember that fear is a normal reaction to a threatening (or perceived dangerous) situation. As you take action, courage will begin to grow inside you, and you will feel stronger, more self-confident, and empowered.

I once knew a young man who worked out daily. Part of his work-out was to jog in the city park. One day as he was jogging he happened upon a Doberman Pinscher that blocked his way. It snarled, baring its sharp, pointed teeth, drooling saliva. The young man knew if he ran the Doberman would outrun him and probably attack. He squarely faced the dog, hunched down in a boxer's stance and said, "Okay, dog, it's you and me. Let's go." The Doberman felt the young man's courage, saw his intention to fight, gave one last growl, and trotted away. This is a very dangerous thing to do, and I would not recommend it myself, but it illustrates the principle of facing your fears.

Your own particular fears may appear like a vicious dog, but once you face them they become gentle puppies. Fear can help us avoid a dangerous situation and should not be ignored, but let's not let fears keep us from doing the things we want to do.

## Waiting for the Big One

*California is the worst place in the world to be buried in. They get them earth-quakes out there. They put you in your box in the ground there, and the earth-quakes keep knocking you around. That way your bones don't get a chance to rest in peace the way they oughta.*

*—Archie Bunker, "All in the Family"*

How can we maintain our positive beliefs and attitudes even in the face of tragedy? What will we do when "The Big One" hits? What is the big one? How will we react? It is of utmost importance to learn how to deal with the "little ones" so that when we are hit with a truly life changing crisis we are prepared to deal with it. According to my colleague, Richard Romano, "If the micro-crises of everyday life get to you, you're toast when the big one hits." One of the best ways to deal with any crisis is through humor. Archie Bunker makes light of a subject that is treated with such seriousness in our culture, and it is serious. But we can lighten things up and not take all of life so seriously. If we can do this we will survive anything. Can you rise daily and do even a 10-minute meditation? You can stay strong even in the face of tragedy if you do this. If we can keep our sense of humor when "bad" things happen to us, we can move on and overcome our grief. Our belief in a loving spiritual being may be shattered when we are hit with bad times, and we may project our fury at God, asking, "How could you let this happen?" We realize from these heartbreaking lessons that no one is immune to pain and suffering, and we can learn and grow from the experience.

Lance Armstrong, in his book, *It's Not About the Bike*, puts it well. "How do you confront your own death? Sometimes I think the blood-brain barrier is more than just physical, it's emotional, too. Maybe there's a protective mechanism in our psyche that prevents us from accepting our mortality unless we absolutely have to."

I agree with Lance. Until I had cancer I mildly glazed over the subject of dying, but never really "believed in my mind" that it pertained to me. Isn't it sad that it took such an event to wake me up? Don't wait until you have a serious illness to wake up to life. Start living now!

My brother-in-law committed suicide, leaving his family shattered. No matter how hard I tried, I simply could not find anything positive that came out of his death. It wasn't until later that I could see things more objectively and come to a different conclusion. There were changes in members of the family that had softened them, made them more compassionate. I had more compassion for others going through the same crisis. And it was during that time that I had my first experience with what I call the "death energy."

My spiritual beliefs had always been strong but had never been tested. When my brother-in-law died, I had the opportunity to witness the fact that the spirit truly does live on after leaving the body. On the night of his funeral I was sleeping soundly when I was awakened by a loud buzzing sound, similar to high tension wires. I did not see anything clearly, but there was an impression of a large body standing in the doorway. The buzzing was intense and I was terrified. I knew instantly that it was my brother-in-law, and I think he was coming to say good-bye, but I was too frightened to do anything except say, "Get out of here, you're scaring me!" The entity disappeared. I would rather have had some other way of testing my spiritual beliefs, but that experience convinced me that the spirit does indeed live on after the body dies.

## Roll Up Your Sleeves and Get to Work

It takes a lot of work to change old beliefs and attitudes and I commend you for attempting this. If you have habitually been a negative thinker, it may take many months to turn that around. Keep going, and never give up. You will reach your goal. Meditate each morning and give thanks each evening. Affirm that you will receive only the best and believe it, and start practicing the art of expectation. Take the time for quiet reflection. Those quiet moments can make all the difference in a busy life. Ask for what you want, believe you will get it, and write an affirmation claiming it. Repeat that affirmation over and over until it gets into your soul. Thought precedes action. What your mind thinks the body follows. When you have setbacks, look at them as opportunities to make you stronger. Remember Weebles? They were toys that always popped back up when you tried to knock them over. "Weebles wobble but they don't fall down." Let this be your motto.

In the movie *Cool Hand Luke*, Paul Newman gets in a rip-roaring fight. He is clearly the loser, but every time he gets knocked down, he gets back up. He won't stay down. Keep that picture in your mind. Every time life knocks you down, get back up. It might take some time if the "punch" is intense, but you can do it. Without some form of belief, either in yourself, God, or something else, life can beat you down.

Lance Armstrong wrote in his book, "Without belief, we would be left with nothing but an overwhelming doom, every single day. And it will beat you.

"I didn't fully see, until the cancer, how we fight every day against the creeping negatives of the world, how we struggle daily against the

---

**Doubt vs. Faith**

*Doubt sees the obstacles,*
*Faith sees the way,*
*Doubt sees the darkest night,*
*Faith sees the day.*
*Doubt dreads to take a step*
*Faith soars on high.*
*Doubt Questions, "Who Believes?"*
*Faith answers, "I."*

—*Author Unknown*

---

slow lapping of cynicism. Dispiritedness and disappointment, these were the real perils of life, not some sudden illness or cataclysmic millennium doomsday. I know now why people fear cancer: because it is a slow and inevitable death, it is the very definition of cynicism and loss of spirit. So, I believed."

Doubt can erase the work you've done, but faith will open doors. It's okay to doubt for a time, to have bad days, and it's at this time that we need to use all the resources we can to get back up. Be easy on yourself in any case, love yourself, and begin to live a life fully in the moment. Worrying about a future that may never happen is a waste of time and energy. Try to stay focused in the present. Be grateful, be happy, and you will be healthy. You will find peace in your life that will stay with you. Believe in yourself and watch the miracles start to happen.

---

So:

- Have you chosen to be happy?
- Have you kept a positive attitude in the face of adversity?
- Do you now see that it is possible to keep a positive attitude in the face of adversity?
- Have you started to change?
- Have you forgiven someone in your life?

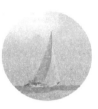

# Plotting Your Course
## Don't Skip Steps

*My philosophy in life, Mildred, is that nothing in life is worth doing unless it can be accomplished with a short cut.*

*—Remington Steele*

Consider the following:

- Do you have enough time in the day to do everything you want to do?
- Do you skip steps or look for a shortcut when doing it?
- Do you feel that you ever waste time?
- Do you ever say, "I don't have enough time for that"?
- Do you often feel rushed?
- Do you have a problem saying no to others?
- Do you pace yourself?

If you nodded while reading any of those, once again, you're not alone. In today's hurried "24/7" society, it's common to feel like you're playing "Beat the Clock." But how often does that hurriedness ultimately cause us trouble? The old cliché says "haste makes waste," and there's more than a kernel of truth to that. Haste does make waste, and that waste can range from something probably not all that tragic—like doing a sloppy job on a project at work or elsewhere—to something as serious as getting in a traffic accident because you were in a hurry to get someplace.

## Take the Time to Do It Right
*If a job's not done right, it's not worth doing.*

—*Old Yankee Saying*

O ne of the most important lessons we can learn in life is to not skip steps. Many of us are in a hurry. We have drive-through banks, drive through pharmacies, I've even heard of drive-through weddings and funerals! We may want to get from Point A to Point B, and we want to get there now! By not skipping steps we can lay a firm foundation so that by the time we get to Point B, we have mastered whatever it is we needed to do to get there. We won't need to look back, go over old stuff, look over our shoulder, or worry that something isn't quite right. We will have taken things one step at a time and we will have arrived at our destination with a sense of purpose and a feeling of accomplishment. By taking the time to do the job right, we can actually avoid some crises.

Think of life as a stairway. You are climbing to the second floor, taking each step one at a time. If you are young, agile, and energetic, you could skip every other step and make it to the second floor in half the time. But what could happen doing it this way? You could trip. You might miss the next step, fall and get hurt. By skipping steps you could actually lose time. If you did manage to skip that step and not trip, it might be worth taking a second look. Was there something important you missed? Was there a lesson you could have learned or a gem you didn't see? Should you take a second look? Will this take more time than if you had just taken that step?

## Not Very Funny
*Patience is a virtue, possess it if you can.*
*Seldom found in women, never in a man.*

—*Old English saying*

Sometimes in the excitement of pursuing our dream, we jump into the deep end of the pool even though we can't swim. We keep right on going anyway, but we may get in over our heads. Being a risk taker, that's exactly how I learned to swim. Sometimes I used that technique in other areas of my life without very good results. When I moved to Saratoga Springs in 1997, I had decided I wanted to be a speaker and thought it would be fun to work with humorists. I walked in to the Humor Project, which hosts an international conference on "Humor and Creativity" every year, and naively asked if they needed any speakers for the spring conference. The secretary asked me if I had a video. "No, not yet." Then she asked me if I had a press package. "No, I don't have one of those either." Very politely she asked me what my program was. "Uh, my program?" "Yes, what's your topic?" Oh, that was easy. "I want to be a motivational speaker." This kind woman gently told me to come back when I had a program and a press package, and then we could talk. It wasn't funny at the time, but now I can see the humor in it.

The expression "putting the cart before the horse" comes to mind when I think of that moment in my life. Talk about skipping steps! Just a few million! I went home, licked my wounds, and set up a plan. My strategy involved joining Toastmasters public speaking group, attending speaker's school and writer's conferences, and reading everything I could about public speaking. Many years and many steps later, I knew I was ready.

## Time Bandits

*Iron rusts from disuse, stagnant water loses its purity and in cold weather becomes frozen: even so does inaction sap the vigors of the mind.*
—*Leonardo da Vinci*

Time. There are so many ways we can waste it. Being diagnosed with cancer gave me a whole new perspective about time, but you don't need cancer to realize you only have a certain amount here on earth. If you don't guard your time and use it wisely, it will slip through your hands like sand in an hourglass.

The definition of "time" is: "A period during which an action, process or condition exists or continues." Learning to manage your time wisely can change your entire outlook on life. The key is to balance daily obligations, work, and fun. I believe it is also important to have time for doing "nothing." Leave days on your calendar blank, with nothing specific to do. Let yourself do something "spur of the moment." By not crowding your schedule with things you *have* to do, you'll have more time for doing things you *want* to do. This way you won't have to "create a crisis" to get out of those things you dislike doing.

I once worked with a woman who was the busiest person I had ever met. She had meetings and business deals, family obligations, and things she "had" to do. She was so busy she didn't have time to think. She seemed to get sick or have accidents quite often. My boss pointed out to me that she didn't allow herself to take time off, so she "created" an illness or accident that provided her with the time she needed to rest and recharge.

Managing time is really about learning to do things more efficiently and eliminating other things altogether. How are you spending your time? Where are you wasting your time? Get a notebook, label it "My Time," and start taking notes. This will help you see what you do with your time. My notebook revealed that I spent most of my time in the kitchen. I love to collect cookbooks from my travels and try different recipes. It seemed like the longer I spent in the kitchen, the more time I could spend there. I determined how much time I wanted to spend cooking and forced myself to stop after that time had elapsed. This was very difficult for me, especially if I hadn't finished what I was doing.

Our world seems to be running full speed ahead, and it is up to us to slow things down. A friend living in Los Angeles told me life was so busy there, he saw a carload of nuns run a red light! When we slow down our lives and keep them in balance, we can be less stressed, less tired, and we'll look and feel better. There seems to be an attitude in our country that if we have idle time, we aren't successful, or we're not doing something right. Don't believe it. Idle time can be spent "recharging the batteries" and used quite effectively.

## Walking the Tightrope of Life

Niagara Falls has long been a vacation destination for honeymooners and families. Daredevils have challenged the mighty falls in barrels and other homemade contraptions, some surviving the hazardous trip over the falls, but many losing their lives and plunging to their deaths as they misjudged the incredible force of the water. Crowds especially loved the tightrope walkers. In 1859 Jean Francis Gravelet, known by his stage name Blondin, took his first trip across the falls. Crowds were awed as he skipped, walked backwards, lay down, turned somersaults, walked on stilts, and even cooked an omelet on a grill he carried with him! At a second performance he held out his hat while sharpshooter John Travis, standing below on the river boat Maid of the Mist, shot a bullet through it. The crowd roared with pleasure.

The key to a successful trip across the tightrope is taking one step at a time and maintaining balance. When walking the tightrope of life, we must take care not to skip steps. The result of skipping steps and losing our balance may not be as catastrophic as a tightrope walker's, but we could still cause ourselves problems. Keeping our balance when life has turned our world upside down may seem impossible, but by keeping to our daily routine, we can maintain equilibrium. We must get enough rest (even if we need to take medication to do so), we must try to eat well (even if we're not hungry), and we must stay in touch with family and friends.

It is especially important to keep a sense of humor. A crisis is never funny, but we can always find some humor in every situation. Laughter has been called "the best medicine," and this is particularly true during times of crisis. Give yourself permission to enjoy life even at the most difficult times. It will help you through almost anything. You'll avoid becoming depressed and you'll be able to get back on track in a much shorter time.

## Quantum Leaps

Unlike a tightrope walker, there could be certain times in our lives that we may skip steps. A mountain top experience, a life threatening illness, death of a loved one, or winning the lottery are experiences that may have a profound effect on us. These experiences allow us to take a quantum leap from one stage of life to another.

Ebenezer Scrooge had such an experience in Charles Dickens' *A Christmas Carol*. Ebenezer is shown, through a dream, how he has evolved into a stingy, grumpy old man. He is also shown his death by a frightening apparition. Seeing the tombstone with his name on it was enough to jolt him into a different reality! When he awakens he is transformed into a caring, kindly gentleman, full of happiness, generosity, and warmth. It is implied that he will spend the rest of his life righting the wrongs he has made.

Ebenezer may have lived happily ever after, but most of us do not. Even after a transforming event in our lives, we will most likely continue to have crises. By experiencing our own pain and suffering, we become more aware of others' pain. We experience life at a much deeper level. The great news is that we also experience joy and love at a much deeper level! Dealing with major crises helps us see smaller ones in perspective. My new philosophy, even when my car engine blew up, is: "If it isn't life threatening, it's not that bad."

---

"I wanted to live, but whether I would or not was a mystery, and in the midst of confronting that fact, even at that moment, I was beginning to sense that to stare into the heart of such a fearful mystery wasn't a bad thing.

"To be afraid is a priceless education. Once you have been that scared, you know more about your frailty than most people, and I think that changes a man.

"I was brought low, and there was nothing to take refuge in but the philosophical: this disease would force me to ask more of myself as a person than I ever had before, and to seek out a different ethic."

—Lance Armstrong, from his book, *It's Not About the Bike.*

## Slow and Steady Wins the Race

*You don't have to do everything, all at once,*
*full force, right away, all the way. Do the next thing.*

—Linus Mundy

Pacing ourselves is one of the ways we can maintain stamina and energy when we are managing our time. Remember the story of the tortoise and the hare? The hare challenged the tortoise to a race. All the animals in the forest came out to watch what would surely be an easy win for the hare. The start and finish lines were marked off, the start signal was given, and off they went. The hare streaked forward at a furious pace, leaving the tortoise in the dust. The tortoise, undaunted, kept going, one foot in front of the other. Further ahead, the hare had gotten a bit tired from his fast pace and decided to take a nap. He had plenty of time before the tortoise ever caught up with him. The tortoise kept on walking. The hare awoke to cheering and howling. "What's going on?" he wondered. He realized the tortoise was at the finish line, and he had no way of catching him. The tortoise had won the race!

Haven't we all rushed off to start something we were really excited about? After working full steam ahead we may get tired, lose our original enthusiasm, and suddenly the project loses its appeal. Wouldn't it be better to pace ourselves like the tortoise? Sure, we can get excited about the job, but if we take it one step at a time, we'll be able to recharge and energize ourselves as we move forward, and not get burned out. We may not have the highs of excitement, but we won't have the lows of disappointment either.

Are you time-oriented or task-oriented? Some people begin a task and don't stop until they are finished. If you are time oriented, you may rush to finish in a certain amount of time. Pace yourself by working hard and then taking a break. You won't feel so burned out, and your job or project will turn out better. Taking a break could include going for a walk or jog, listening to music, meditating, reading, taking a short nap, or doing some stretching and breathing exercises. If the job or activity stretches over a year or two, make sure you plan a vacation sometime during that period.

Is it difficult for you to say "no"? Many times we'll say "yes" to a favor or a special project before we think it through. Do we really want to do this? What does it involve? How much time will it take? Think it through carefully before you say yes. A good rule is to tell people you always sleep on any decision you make. This gives you a breather and some time to think about it. Don't let

## 10 Tips for Managing Your Time

1. Avoid tackling too many jobs at once.
2. Try to estimate how long each job will take.
3. Don't spend time on trivial things to avoid doing the important jobs.
4. Learn how to say no gracefully, tactfully, and firmly.
5. Set deadlines. Set reasonable goals so you don't get discouraged.
6. Take a break. After each hour of work take five to 10 minutes to refresh.
7. Use travel and waiting time wisely. Bring a book, review your time planner.
8. Be aware of time wasters. Talking on the phone, watching too much TV, video games.
9. Avoid procrastinating. Keep moving, give yourself that extra push.
10. Notice and use daily cycles of energy. If you're a morning person, do your most difficult work then.

people pressure you into making a decision until you are ready to give them an honest and well thought out answer.

Sometimes we're flattered when someone asks us to help out on an important project. We may have the opportunity of working with people we respect at an interesting job. A few weeks before I started my chemotherapy treatments I was asked to be the campaign manager for a friend's election in Saratoga Springs. I said "yes," but pointed out right up front that I would soon begin treatment for recurring cancer, but that I would help out in any way I could. About the same time another friend, a successful jazz musician, asked me to help market his CDs. I was feeling good at the time, but once I started my treatments, all that changed. I realized the amount of work and time involved in each job was too much for me. Sadly, I had to leave both jobs and take time to heal and get my energy back. Happily, my candidate won and the musician sold plenty of CDs.

That experience taught me to think through the amount of time and effort involved in any job I agreed to do. I also learned that if I get in over my head, it's okay. I just need to know when to let go and walk away. Learning how to admit a mistake and being courageous enough to step down are admirable traits.

How many times do we say "yes" because we can't think of a good way to say "no" when we are put on the spot? Take a notebook or journal and spend some time thinking of ways to say no. Your answers should be honest, legitimate, and polite. There may be a day in the future when you can say yes. One possible answer could be, "Gee, I'd love to help you with your project, but I'm really swamped right now. Why don't you give me a call in six months and we can see what's going on then?" Write out your answers and practice them a few times so you'll remember them.

## The Elephant Walk
> *I skate to where the puck is going to be, not where it is.*
> —*Wayne Gretzky*

Sometimes the "steps of life" seem ungainly and awkward. Things do not always happen perfectly. Life does not give us staircases with landings placed at just the right spots. When I was attending the University of Rhode Island, there was a set of stairs leading down to the cafeteria. We fondly called it the "elephant walk." The stairs were built too wide to be able to take them one step at a time, and too narrow to take them two steps at a time. The students decided the steps were just the right distance for an elephant's gait, thus the name "elephant walk."

Life gives us plenty of "elephant walks," but we still can't skip the steps. When events are thrust upon us, unwanted and unexpected, we may have to deal with them immediately. If we have to delay dealing with the crisis because it is too overwhelming at the moment, we can compartmentalize it in a section of our minds I call a "neutral zone." Things in the neutral zone remain there until we have the strength and support we need to deal with them. It is important to eventually deal with it, or we may never return to it and it could cause us trouble in the future.

I found myself walking an "elephant walk" when I moved to New York. My expectations were to start a new life and career, buy a beautiful home, prepare my children for college, and enjoy the opportunities abounding in Saratoga Springs. Instead I got three recurrences of cancer over the next two years and finally had to do chemotherapy every week for 15 months. I wanted to skip steps and get a job even though I knew working would slow the healing process. I had to stay home and recuperate, living off savings. It was one of the most difficult times of my life.

## Dropping the Anchor

What could cause us to skip steps? Anxiety over money can be extremely stressful, and, as in my case, caused a lot of angst. The winter I couldn't work was one of the snowiest on record in upstate New York, and high oil prices contributed to a high outflow of money! The cost of daily living has escalated to alarming heights. Taking care of elderly parents and sending our children to college have become financial burdens. When my daughter found out how much it cost per year for higher education, she realized why parents turn white when it's time to send their children to college. Many people cannot save for a catastrophe because minimum wage does not mean a living wage. Yogi Berra was right when he said, "A nickel ain't worth a dime anymore." When my sister and I compared the costs of nursing homes for our mother, we realized it might be cheaper to hire a private nurse to take care of her. Money concerns could cause us to take an extra job, go back to work too soon after an operation, or take out a loan we can't repay. Any of these could cause a new crisis.

> "Always when I woke up, I had the feeling which I am sure must be natural to all of us, a joy in being alive. I don't say you feel it consciously—you don't—but there you are, you are alive, and you open your eyes, and here is another day; another step, as it were, on your journey to an unknown place, that very exciting journey which is your life. Not that it is necessarily going to be as exciting as a life, but it will be exciting to you because it is your life. That is one of the great secrets of existence, enjoying the gift of life that has been given to you."
> —*Agatha Christie from her autobiography*

## Take Life One Step at a Time

By not skipping steps we'll be more organized, better prepared, and emotionally ready when crisis hits. We'll have laid a strong foundation for those times in our lives that could be overwhelming. We can also help others going through troubles, and our help will be greatly appreciated. It is important not to skip steps along the way and to realize the important things in life. I'd like to share a story with you I found on the Internet:

## "The Importance of Rocks"

A philosophy professor stood before his class and had some items in front of him. When the class began, wordlessly he picked up an empty glass jar and proceeded to fill it with rocks, right to the top. He then asked the students if the jar was full. They agreed that it was.

The professor then picked up a box of pebbles and poured them into the jar. He shook the jar lightly. The pebbles, of course, rolled into the open areas between the rocks. The students laughed. He asked them again if the jar was full. They agreed that yes, it was. The professor then picked up a container of sand and poured it into the jar. Of course, the sand filled up everything else.

"Now," said the professor, "I want you to recognize that this is your life. The rocks are the important things—your family, your partner, your health, your children—anything that is so important to you that if it were lost, you would be nearly destroyed. The pebbles represent things like your job, your house, your car. The sand is everything else. The small stuff. If you put the sand or the pebbles into the jar first, there is no room for the rocks. The same goes for your life. If you spend all your energy and time on the small stuff, material things, you will never have room for the things that are most important.

Pay attention to the things that are critical in your life. Play with your children. Take time to get medical checkups. Take your partner out dancing. There will always be time to go to work, clean the house, give a dinner party and fix the disposal."

Take care of the rocks first—the things that really matter. Set your priorities. The rest is just pebbles and sand.

---

Now:

- Have you made more time to do the things you want?
- Have you skipped any steps?
- Have you stopped wasting time?
- Have you stopped saying, "I don't have time for that?"
- Do you still feel rushed?
- Have you started saying no?
- Are you pacing yourself?

# Sirens, Mermaids, and Monsters of the Deep

## Think Creatively

*We are all faced with a series of great opportunities brilliantly disguised as impossible situations.*

—*Chuck Swindol*

---

Ask yourself the following:

- Do you believe you are a creative thinker?
- Do you believe you have to be born "gifted" to be creative?
- Can you think of ways to have fun in a "serious" situation?
- Do you know how to find creative ideas by mind mapping?
- Do you know Leonardo da Vinci's seven principles of creativity?
- Do you meditate daily?

It may seem odd to think of creativity as being an essential component to crisis management, but being able to think "outside the box" or in unorthodox ways is an essential component of your arsenal of coping tools. From being able to see hidden solutions to problems to simply not taking insignificant things too seriously, creative thinking can really come in handy.

---

## Revolution!

Quiet filled the darkness. My ears strained for the sound that had woken me. There. Loud booming. Ferocious in its power. Fireworks? No, too deep, too angry. Guns? Artillery? Impossible. Then what was that noise? I bolted upright as the phone rang. It was my downstairs neighbor, Antonio.

"Don't go outside, Kim, they're having a revolution out there, a real bloodbath." Revolution? In Portugal? Bloodbath? Since it was 6:00 in the morning, there was little chance of me venturing outside, but my stomach knotted up when I realized that the sounds that had awakened me were indeed dangerous. "As soon as it's light we'll see what's going on. I'll call you later." Antonio and Lella lived two floors below mine and were invaluable resources for me. A Portuguese/Spanish couple attending the University of Lisbon, they had befriended my (now ex-) husband and me when we moved to Portugal. Wanting to practice their English, they spoke it at any opportunity, and translated for us whenever we needed help.

Sleep was impossible. I unlatched the glass door leading to the veranda and curiously poked my head outside. A faint rumbling from Avenida da Roma suggested thunder, but I realized it was the subway. City streets normally filled with honking, impatient drivers speeding to work were empty. Usual throngs of shoppers buying fresh bread and the day's dinner were nowhere to be seen. No 747s roaring over the top of the apartment building across the street. No "pineapple carts" filled with fresh fruit buzzing along the back streets. No fishmongers pushing cod, the catch of the day. No uniformed Portuguese children pushing and laughing and teasing each other on their way to school. Not even the newspaper man singing, "O Jornal, senora?" The silence was deafening, creepy. Even the ubiquitous pigeons sensed danger and lay quiet, roosting in the tops of the high rises.

The phone rang again. Antonio suggested we venture out to investigate and see if any stores were open. We crept along the city streets, occasionally passing a lone walker, and ducking "Avisos," flyers promoting a favorite political party, tossed up and swept along with the damp chilly breeze of the early morning.

Thankfully, a supermarket was open. Once in the store, however, we were caught up in utter chaos. Panic-stricken Portuguese grabbed anything edible from shelves already picked over. We followed their lead, snatching bread, milk, packages of dried soup powder and cereal, running out of luck as we scurried down the aisles. Pushing and shoving, we made our way to the check-out aisle, counted out our escudos, and bagged our groceries. Between the four of us, we had managed to fill four bags. Flushed with our success, we started back home. The streets were still empty.

Holding up his hand, Antonio yelled for us to stop. "Quick, run in here!" he shouted, pushing us into a narrow cobbled alley. The look of concern on his face frightened me, and hearing an unfamiliar sound drawing closer to our hiding place, I suddenly understood his urgency.

Tanks rumbled down the street as we pushed back against the crumbling cement wall in the alleyway. Soldiers stood atop, rifles held ready. Shaking, we ran to the end of the alley, praying we reached our street before the tanks. Breaking into a full-fledged run, we cut down another alley, around the corner and finally reached our apartment building. Antonio fumbled with the key as he unlocked the door. It took us a full minute to catch our breath. Swallowing hard, we stared at each other and ran up the stairs into Antonio and Lella's apartment.

As soon as we shut the door, we heard the tanks roaring down the street. Horrified, Antonio let down the heavy outdoor blinds and darkness filled the apartment. Lella switched on the overhead light. No one spoke.

Antonio turned on the radio after lunch. There had been a military coup, and the dictator Salazar had been overthrown. So far no one knew who had power. We sat in Antonio and Lellas' apartment the rest of the day making small talk, finding some comfort in each other's company. Tanks continued creaking and clanking along the city streets and we heard sporadic bursts of gunfire throughout the day. My stomach was still in knots. As darkness dropped over the city we left the warmth and comfort of my friends' apartment and walked up the two flights to ours. I spent the night tossing and turning, dreaming of soldiers with huge machine guns firing at the lovely old tiled buildings in downtown Lisbon.

A few days later I tried to call home. All the international lines were busy, so I didn't get a call through until the next day. By then things had gotten somewhat worse in Lisbon, as there was some resistance to the takeover. My family began to devise some rather creative means for an escape from Portugal. It just wasn't safe for Americans anymore they insisted, especially if the Communists took control. "Get out of Portugal!" they shouted. "Take a train up to the border and sneak into Spain or France." Were the trains even running? What about all those soldiers with machine guns? Were they only in Lisbon? Where would we find food? Would we have enough money?

The Portuguese revolution in 1974 turned out to be relatively peaceful, and we flew out of Lisbon a week or so later. Soldiers stood at attention holding loaded machine guns as we boarded our plane, and I could hear loud yelling in the background. The situation was far from safe, but I knew we would return to Lisbon as soon as things settled down.

## Creative Solutions

> *The absence of alternatives clears the mind marvelously.*
> —*Henry Kissinger*

Living through a revolution was both frightening and exciting. Frightening because of the feeling of loss of control, fear of the unknown, and fear of bodily harm. Exciting because of the challenge to make it through a potentially life threatening situation. How could I escape from one foreign country to another? How could I survive in a city overtaken by tanks and armed soldiers? Where would I get my food? Where would I find shelter if the city was attacked?

When we are faced with a threat to our lives, we get in touch with our souls. It is at this level we are able to find creative answers to our questions as we connect with the Divine, the Creator of all things, all intelligence. It is here we find the information we are looking for. The popularity of the show "Survivor" validates this urge in us to use these latent talents. Our minds are pitted against other minds. We must think on our feet. We must survive! (And perhaps win a million dollars.) Paintball "wars" have long been popular as well. My daughter participated in one of these adventures and loved every minute of it. She has a sweet, passive Libra personality, and it was interesting how much she enjoyed the challenge. How often do you use your creative talents in an exciting, challenging way? You don't need a revolution, a trip to the Australian outback, or a paintball war. You can find your own ways of tapping into that part of you which creates.

Thinking creatively can be learned. You do not have to be born an Albert Einstein or a Leonardo da Vinci to be creative. Many think creative people have a rare artistic talent, had parents who encouraged their creativity, or had an education in the fine arts. Others think you have to be right brained rather than left brained. Many of us also think that being creative means being an artist, a musician, or a writer. None of this is so. You don't need any of these things to be creative. All you need is the desire and the will. If you can open your mind, feel with your heart, empty your mind, and let go, you can be creative. Think of your life as a canvas, and paint a masterpiece using your own creative talents. You have them, you just may not have realized it. Creating your life artistically will bring you the excitement and enthusiasm that may be lacking in your life. Get excited! Get out the paintbrushes and paints of your mind and get started! Begin with the mundane things in your life and bring them to life. Dig into that majestic place deep in your soul that is longing to give you a love and vitality for life. Dive into the depths of your fantastic mind and discover just how wonderful you really are!

Once you begin to live your life creatively, some interesting things begin to happen. You won't take things so personally when people criticize you. You'll realize they are simply reacting to something in you that may be missing in their lives, and they may be jealous of your new zest for living. You won't worry about what others think because you won't be thinking about them. You won't compare yourself to others and find yourself lacking, because you aren't lacking anything and never were. You will begin to think more positively, and any destructive thinking habits will melt away as you take better care of yourself, learn to appreciate who you are, and really start to love yourself. You will begin to rely on your own common sense and experiences in life to guide you. You'll listen to advice from others, take what you can use, and discard the rest. What benefits you'll reap! You will have increased self esteem, and you'll be more assertive, happy, and peaceful. You'll have a joy and excitement towards life, so when you are blind-sided by the inevitable crises, you'll bounce back much faster because you won't hit bottom so hard.

Why don't more people think and behave creatively? The most obvious reason is that it takes effort and change. Many people feel comfortable exactly where they are. It is difficult and frightening to leave our comfort zones. If we are to be more creative, we must be different and stand out. This may be too difficult for some. Those who do not live a creative life may be afraid to take risks. Taking risks may feel like taking a Bungee jump. Yes, there is risk when we step out of our comfort zone, but isn't it exhilarating when we do?

One of the greatest risks I have ever taken was the year I had to do a course of chemotherapy and decided to write this book. I had to live off my savings and accept monetary help from my mother (which really healed our relationship). It was a year I held my breath and prayed nothing would need repairing in my home, the kids wouldn't break any bones or need surgery, and I would be well enough to complete the manuscript. Things did break in my home, my car needed major repairs, my daughters were in a car accident and totaled their car, and in one week I got pneumonia, an infected toe, and three cavities! Yet I managed to survive and get the book written. I kept asking myself: How am I going to keep everything going, pay my bills, write a book, do chemo, visit colleges, prepare for my daughter's high school graduation, and have some fun? It was great for testing my ability to think creatively. It was a year of reaching deep inside myself, asking for lots of help, and learning to trust God to be there for my children and me. Just when I needed money to pay the oil bill, I received a check in the mail from an unexpected source. Just when I needed some emotional support, a friend would call and tell me she was thinking about me. I learned to trust and to be able to take greater risks.

## Don't Get Older, Get Better!
*When you're through changing, you're through.*
—*Bruce Barton*

As we grow older, it seems we become much less creative. How do we lose our creativity? Little by little society strips us of our childlike freshness. Families, companies, schools, and religious institutions encourage group thinking, and anyone who tries to break the mold is considered a troublemaker. Reason and logic are rewarded in our schools, whereas humor, intuition, and fancy are frowned upon. Many of our children who do not fit the mold of our educational system have been labeled uncooperative, or diagnosed with Attention Deficit Disorder. The present trend of giving medication to "help" these children is somewhat alarming. Do they really have a "problem," or are they acting outside the mold? Should we expect every child in the United States to learn the same way? Are we churning out "cookie cutter kids"?

Businesses and corporations claim to be "innovative," yet are they really? An innovative and creative worker would question tradition, challenge the rules, suggest new ways of doing things, tell the truth, and generally appear disruptive to the rest of the employees. Have you ever known someone who was truly innovative? Was he considered a troublemaker in the firm? Did she keep her job? Was he labeled a "kook"? I love the innovative genius of Southwest Airlines. Their methods fly in the face of "normal." Taking risks, the CEO dared to do something completely different from any other airline, and consequently Southwest has become one of the most successful airlines in the United States. On one trip, our flight attendant described safety procedures and then announced, "My daughter will now serve you refreshments." Hiring members of the same family in other airlines is unthinkable. Employees are encouraged to use their spirit of creativity, and on another flight the pilot actually came out of the cockpit and introduced himself. Other flight attendants have told poetry, sung, and told jokes. How refreshing!

We may sabotage our own creativity for fear of losing our jobs, or may be afraid we might fail if we try something we've never done before. We may be just plain lazy, lack self-motivation, or have become stale. We think, it's better if I just stay quiet and not make waves. What are the consequences of making changes in my life? Things really aren't that bad. If I rock the boat I may be sorry. What's the use anyway?

Yet your imagination can be your greatest ally. Do you ever complain about your life? Do you sit around and mope or get crabby about the state of things? Are you ever bored? Have you lost the joy of living? Living creatively can change your perspective on life. You can turn around the complaints and find things to be thankful for. You can change crabby thoughts to humorous ones. You can bury boredom and find fun in even the worst state of events. You can rediscover the joy of living, even when things appear negative.

During my nine-year "medical odyssey," I had many procedures and operations that required me to stay in the hospital. Sleeping in a hospital bed tethered to an IV bag, smelling foul and noxious odors, humiliated by my behind showing every time I got out of bed, and listening to "the screams of the tortured" was not my idea of fun. Taking a cue from my father, a true creative genius who could take any situation and have fun with it, I pulled off a caper he would have been proud of.

My room was labeled "private." That was a joke. A cardboard wall divided one large room into two, allowing me to hear every sound made by the patient in the next room. One night the nurses brought an elderly woman back from the operating room. Their method of bringing the woman around was to turn the TV on *loud*. It seemed like a stressful way to be woken up, and the truly annoying thing was that while it did not work on the patient, it was working on me! I know I could have called the nurse and explained that the TV was keeping me awake, but I had other plans. Giggling and feeling mischievous, I savored being my father's daughter that night.

Tiptoeing from my bed to the doorway, I poked my head out of the door to make sure the coast was clear. In my mind I played the theme song from "Mission: Impossible." With my back pressed against the wall, I sneaked along the corridor into the old woman's room and turned the TV down to a whisper. I flew back to my room, jumped into bed, and pulled the covers up to my neck, pretending to be asleep. Ahhh, peace and quiet.

Not for long. Half an hour later I heard the squeak of the nurse's shoes in the old lady's room. My heart sank. I gave the nurse a full five minutes to return to the nurse's station before tiptoeing back to the old woman's room.

Again, "Mission: Impossible" music playing in my head, checking to make sure the coast was clear, I sneaked into her room again and turned the TV down to a whisper. I was in my bed with the covers up before anyone was the wiser. Sometime later I was woken by loud voices of a man and woman arguing. It was the TV. I pictured the nurse scratching her head trying to figure out how that TV kept turning itself down. I chuckled, waited 10 minutes, and repeated my mission.

The next thing I knew it was morning. The TV was silent. I had won! Smiling all day, I sent good wishes to the elderly woman for a full recovery. I waited eagerly for the nurse to complain to the electrician on call about the television in room 507, and wished I could hear him saying, "I can't find a thing wrong with it!"

This may not be your idea of fun, but it gave me a good laugh while in the hospital. The message here is, find the fun in a situation and go with it. We don't have to be crabby about anything. If someone at work is giving you a hard time, make up a goofy name for them and a cartoon character that fits their personality. Draw a whole comic book scenario of the situation, and next time you see that person, think of them by that cartoon name. Never, under any circumstances, tell them about this. It is solely for you and should never be shared with anyone. The idea is not to hurt someone or make fun of them. It is merely for you to be able to get beyond a difficult situation.

### This is Your Brain on Drugs. Any Questions?

*I used to think the human brain was the most fascinating part of the body.*
*Then I realized—what is telling me that?*

—*Comedian Emo Philips*

Remember the commercial a few years ago about drugs and our brain? The first scene showed us an egg being broken into a frying pan. "This is your brain," the announcer said. The next scene showed the egg being fried. "This is your brain on drugs. Any questions?" The ad was very effective. It made us appreciate our brains and urged us not to abuse them.

The human brain is the most remarkable and amazing organ in our bodies. (Yes, I know, what is telling me that?) No one has really explored fully its complexities. The more it is studied the more fascinated we become with it! Our brains contain about one million million (1,000,000,000,000) brain cells. We have heard that most people use only 10% of their brains. Does anyone really know exactly how much of our brain power there is and how much we actually use? I believe we rarely use our brains to their fullest capacity. We can actually increase our brain power as we age, and it's nice to know that there's one part of the body that can keep getting better as we get older. All it takes is a bit of effort. We can do exercises that increase our memories, our learning capacities, and our creative potential, even as we grow old.

Nobel Prize winner Roger Sperry popularized the terms right- and left-brained. Sperry discovered that in most cases, the left part of the brain processes logical, analytical thinking, while the right side of the brain processes imaginative, visual, perceptual thinking. The left and right sides of the brain share and communicate their views by way of a nerve bundle called the corpus callosum. The two sides work cooperatively. A musician uses the left side of the brain while reading the music and keeping the beat, while the right side handles tone, melody, and expression. In the creative process, the left side likes all the facts and the right side likes all the ideas. Using the two sides of the brain in a balanced way, we can create just about anything we put our minds to.

## Mind Mapping

*I try not to have any ideas. It only leads to complications.*
*—Johnny Fever in "WKRP in Cincinnati"*

A tremendously powerful method of bringing the two sides of the brain together is a process called *mind mapping*. It's a method for generating ideas, organizing them, and putting it all together. It was conceived by Tony Buzan and inspired by the method in which Leonardo da Vinci took notes. Leonardo's note taking consisted of a central theme surrounded by ideas and thoughts, key words, and illustrations. Mind mapping can be used for setting goals, daily planning, and problem solving. It trains you to be a more balanced thinker because the natural thinking process involves impressions, key words, and images, which come into the mind while recalling information. Other names for this method are Idea Tree, Spoke Diagram, Thought Web, and Clustering Diagram.

It's important to write down our ideas so we don't forget what we want to do. Using the Mind Map technique, diaries, photographs, journals, books, and documentaries helps us remember. The Mind Map is great because it is compact, and many ideas can be listed on one page. Looking at the ideas you have created can help generate other ideas. It is a long-term tool. You can set it aside for a while, then come back and generate even more ideas.

My daughter needed some direction for her guitar playing. I explained how mind mapping worked and suggested she try it to set some goals. She

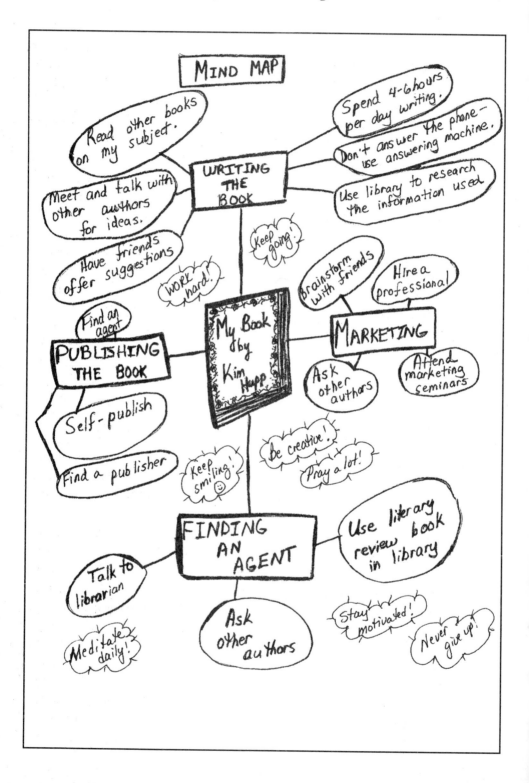

wanted to play the guitar so well it would bring listeners to tears. How could she get to this point? Using the mind mapping technique, she came up with several ideas. Mapping out the plan included talking to both present and past guitar teachers, buying guitar music, practicing "until her fingers bled," and listening to great guitar players. She now had some direction and could begin implementing an action plan.

Mind mapping illustrates the brain in action. The basic structural unit of the brain is the neuron. Each of our billions of neurons branches out from a center called the nucleus. Each branch, or dendrite, is covered with little nodes called dendritic spines. As we think, electrochemical "information" jumps across the tiny gap between spines. This junction is called a synapse. Our thinking is a function of a vast network of synaptic patterns. We can learn seven facts per second, every second for the rest of our lives, and still have plenty of room to learn more. Our brains are also able to make virtually unlimited synaptic connections of potential patterns of thought.

A Mind Map is a graphic expression of these natural patterns of the brain. Charles Darwin, Michelangelo, Mark Twain, and Leonardo da Vinci took notes in much the same way as the brain works. Their note-taking styles feature a branching, brain-like, organic structure filled in with sketches, creative doodles, and key words. Try doing some mind mapping of your own! What is a current problem or goal you would like to work on? Choose a central theme, such as "Writing my first book." Draw a picture of the book and use that as your central theme. Have fun with it! The sky is the limit for ideas on how to get that book written, edited, published, and sold. Once you have the ideas, come up with an action plan to bring them to fruition. Go for the gold and get it done. You can do it!

We can all strive to live a life with more artistic expression. We don't need to actually paint, play music, or write books like da Vinci, but we can create a life based on his principles. What a challenge! When was the last time you opened your heart and really *felt* something? Does your soul feel free or locked up? Have you ever asked about something for the sheer joy of learning something new? How often do you ask, "What if...?" We have much to learn from the great artists. How sad that when our schools cut programs, the first to go are the arts. The arts allow us to get in touch with our souls. When our children come home from school we should wonder, "What questions did you *ask* today?" instead of questioning what they *learned*. Living creatively infuses us with an insatiable quest for knowledge and for the ultimate questions in life: "Why are we here?" "What is my purpose in life?" "How can I give of myself?"

## Leonardo's Seven Principles of Creativity

Leonardo da Vinci lived by seven principles of creativity:

1. The first was an insatiable curiosity for life and a never ending quest for continuous learning.

2. He had a commitment to test knowledge through experience, persistence, and a willingness to learn from mistakes. He was never afraid to make mistakes and actually welcomed them so he could learn even more.

3. He believed in continuously refining the senses, especially sight, and believed this was a means to increase experience.

4. He had a willingness to embrace ambiguity, paradox, and uncertainty.

5. He believed in "whole brain" thinking, and developed a balance between science and art, logic and imagination. He used both his left brain and right brain in a balanced way.

6. He also practiced the cultivation of grace, fitness, and poise.

7. Finally, he had a recognition of, and appreciation for, the interconnectedness of all things and all phenomena that happened in the world.

Perhaps if students learned to love the great masters, they would learn love instead of violence.

We can choose role models to help us. Do you have a hero in your life? Queen Elizabeth I was a great leader, and in the movie *Elizabeth* we can witness some of her methods of leadership. Leonardo da Vinci was a genius and shows us how to use the mind mapping technique, for engineering as well as art. Mark Twain was a gifted writer. The mayor of New York City in 2001 was Rudolph Giuliani, who proved himself a strong and caring leader during the World Trade Center terrorist attacks. Princess Diana, my personal favorite, showed us her human side, allowing us to see that she was vulnerable and could be hurt like anyone else, yet kept her sense of dignity and honor. In the movie *Chocolat*, the heroine offers the cruel mayor a glass of tonic instead of vengeance after he destroys her window display and gets sick from gorging on the chocolate. We can learn from all of them.

"Anti role models" can also teach us what not to do. My Grandma Floyd was the best teacher on how not to raise children. She was taught the "proper" way of childrearing as a nanny for wealthy families, but unfortunately this included verbal and physical abuse. Although she thought she was doing the right thing, it was not a healthy way to raise children. We all know leaders, teachers, and politicians who were less than great. Who was your worst teacher? Your worst boss? Think about what made them so terrible to you and try not to repeat it. Learn from their mistakes.

Most people don't realize just how gifted they really are. Have you ever asked someone "What are you good at?" and they give you a blank stare? Everyone is good at *something*. You may not think you are gifted. You are. You may not think anyone needs you. They do. You are unique, like no one who has come before you or will come after you. No one else can speak with your wondrous voice, smile your beautiful smile, or shine your wondrous light. Use your gifts. The world needs them and you.

## Start Using Your Senses

We can start today to become more creative by using our senses. Open your heart to the magnificent sights, the wondrous sounds, the tender touch, scrumptious tastes, and aromatic smells that are all part of daily living. How sad that we become immune to the wonder of our senses. We cut ourselves off to defend against deafening city noises, the pain of rejection from human touch, noxious odors, poisoned food, and frightening news clips. Yet wondrous beauty is all around us.

Leonardo da Vinci lamented that the average human "looks without seeing, listens without hearing, touches without feeling, eats without tasting, moves without physical awareness, inhales without awareness of odor or fragrance, and talks without thinking." Isn't it amazing how some things never change? How many of us are guilty of the same? Start today to become more aware of the world around you by using your senses. Find the childish wonder that was lost and dulled by the passage of time and by the pain and difficulty of life. Fill your heart with love and laughter, lifting the defensive walls you have built around you. Your life will take on a new dimension you never dreamed possible. Ask yourself, "What is the most beautiful thing I have ever seen?" "What is the sweetest sound I have ever heard?" Imagine a sublimely delicious taste, the softest touch, the most delectable aroma. Cast aside your fears. Your senses, the very essence of your being, cannot hurt you.

## Silence is Golden

*Better to remain silent and be thought a fool,*
*than to speak out and remove all doubt.*

—*Abraham Lincoln*

Using our senses to be more creative is easy and fun. The most important sense to Leonardo da Vinci was sight. He wrote, "...the eye encompasses the beauty of the whole world." Have you ever looked at the world through an artist's eye? Try this exercise to help you "see" better.

Look at something close to you, then change your focus to the farthest horizon. Pick out something specific and focus on it for a few seconds, then bring your focus back to close up. Focus on the horizon again, this time picking out something different. Do this for five minutes. What did you notice?

Another exercise is to find a picture or plan to watch a sunset. Describe it in detail. Note colors, shapes, ways the sun moves, the way clouds are shaped. Really experience the sunset. Doesn't this make you feel the wonder of our world?

One lovely autumn morning in October, I was listening to a talk by Sister Anne Bryan Smollin titled, "God Knows You're Stressed." She said that one way to decrease stress was to stay connected, and she suggested smiling and keeping eye contact. A blind woman came up to her after her talk and suggested there was a third way to stay connected, and that was through touch. Sister Anne agreed, and sighed, lamenting the fact that we are becoming a society that is raising children paranoid of being touched. Leonardo revered sight, but let us not forget healthy touch. Have you ever had a massage? Slowly the stereotype of sleazy massage parlors is changing, and qualified massage therapists are working in offices all over the country. Some people might be uncomfortable removing their clothes for a massage, but there are many different types of massage where that is not necessary. I received an incredible back massage with all my clothes on from a massage therapist at a cancer survivors outing. Try a chair massage offered as a promotion at health conventions. *Reiki* is becoming popular, and I had the opportunity to try it. I felt completely relaxed afterwards, and all the practitioner did was touch different parts of my back and shoulders, and I didn't have to remove one article of clothing. If you are thinking about trying massage, I highly recom-

## Mind Your Creativity

Never underestimate your capabilities to solve a problem creatively. Try tapping into the Universal Mind to help with a problem, but if you would rather try to tackle it yourself, use the following four steps.

1. Identify the problem. Sometimes we see the results of a problem, but the original source is something else. When my daughter was having difficulty practicing her harp, I thought she was becoming bored with her music. The real problem was that she was having trouble with her boyfriend.

2. After identifying the true problem, use the mind mapping technique to find as many solutions as you can.

3. Analyze and choose solutions to solve the problem.

4. Implement the solutions. If the first one doesn't work, try another one until you find one that works.

mend it. Make sure you see a qualified massage therapist who has a good reputation.

To increase your appreciation of sounds, try this exercise. Once or twice each day, take a few moments to pause and just listen to the sounds around you. You may hear the loudest noises first, but keep listening until you hear the softest noises. Finally, listen to the silence. Let silence be a theme for the day, and notice what it feels like to be in a place of complete silence.

Smells can bring you right back to a certain place in time. The smell of balsam pine trees brings me right back to the first Christmas I spent in Lisbon, Portugal. There wasn't enough money to buy decorations, so I took the trolley to the business district of the city where merchants were selling Christmas trees. I picked up several small branches that had been cut off the trees, and made a lovely spray and decorated it with ribbons and tinsel. It was one of my fondest memories! What aromas trigger memories for you?

As you awaken your senses, you may suddenly come face to face with the unknown. You may be opening your mind to deeper questions about life and death, and this can trigger some unexpected fears. The unknown can be quite daunting and frightening, but keeping your mind open in the face of the unknown and uncertainty is the single most powerful way you can open your creative potential. Areas of knowledge you never knew existed will open up for you, and you'll be excited by the innovative ideas that will spring forth from you!

## Growing Rocks in New England

I was able to use this creative thinking process in a way that saved me money. I was living in Massachusetts in the 1980s, which made me an official "Yankee." The stereotype is that Yankees are distrustful, so they hide money under their mattresses, bury their silverware in the backyard, and only do business with people they know. Like just about all stereotypes, these are untrue, but speaking as a Yankee, when people say Yankees are cheap, there is a kernel of truth in that, although I prefer the word "frugal."

Rocks have been said to grow in New England, and while living there I had the opportunity to witness such a phenomenon. A bump appeared in my driveway one day, and being a rather small bump, I ignored it. The bump continued to grow, and two years later it was large enough to hit the oil pan of my car. I had no extra money at that time to have the rock removed, and I was also being frugal, so I tried "tapping into the Universal Mind" and asked for a solution to my problem. Not really expecting an answer, I was thrilled when, "out of the blue," a thought struck me. The rock was technically on town property, as it was within three feet of the street. Town hall verified this, and reluctantly sent a crew to remove the rock after I suggested that it would cost them less to remove it than to repair every car that used my driveway. The cost to me? Nothing! Jubilantly, I celebrated the great mind of the Universe.

## Be Flexible

Being flexible is important when solving problems and dealing with life. You may have to "switch gears" in the middle of something, but being flexible reduces much emotional angst. You will be able to respond to the unexpected at a moment's notice, and this could prove invaluable in many situations. Also remember that you are in charge of your own creativity, and you should ignore any advice that does not pertain to you. If it rings true, use it, if not, discard it. Use your creativity and flexibility to work for you, not against you.

One summer I received a scholarship to attend the International Women's Writing Guild Conference held at Skidmore College in Saratoga Springs, New York. I had a bad case of writer's block, and I was excited about attending workshops dedicated to breaking through the blocks. The conference lasted all week, but the particular workshop I wanted was on a Monday. I had a doctor's appointment that day, as I had started my chemotherapy treatments, and when the nurse informed me I had to have a blood transfusion ASAP, I was infuriated. Transfusions are painless, but take about six hours. I had been looking forward to that workshop and was sorely disappointed that I had to miss it. I realized I had to be flexible in this instance, and used the time writing instead of sulking. I attended an evening session and got some notes from the day's lecture, so all was not lost. I saved myself the stress of getting upset by using that "negative" energy to write. It actually helped me break through my block!

Imagination and creativity are crucial for success in life. You will be able to see opportunity in situations where non-creative people see insurmountable problems. You will be able to create positive from negative. You will turn weaknesses into strengths. Best of all, you will turn worries into solved problems! There is an old saying, "When the going gets tough, the tough get going." and "Winners never quit and quitters never win." But some of us don't have the strength of character, you might be saying. How can we grow tough if we have always been a "wimp"? First, you must be motivated. If you really want to be tough and strong, you can. You must be determined. You must persevere. Ask for help if you need to. Pray without ceasing. Never give up. Keep going. You have a strength you never knew you had, just reach into your soul and find it. It is there.

What if you're living a comfortable life? You're happy with the way things are, so why bother living a more creative life? Think of this. What if you could be living a *better* way? Have you thought of all the alternatives? Is there something that you have overlooked that might be more interesting, more exciting, more loving? Are all the people in your life happy?

Living creatively helps us stay up to date in an ever-changing world. We are now in the digital and computer age, and even that is changing at a dramatic pace. Change can be exciting and refreshing. Promoting a business is difficult and creative ideas are a must in order to be successful. How are you going to pay for college? Are you living within your means? Creative thinking can help you in many different areas of your life.

## Little Gremlins (Floydian Slips)

As soon as you start planning and living a more creative life, something happens. A voice begins to speak to you. Some call it the "Voice of Judgment" or the "Voice of Reason." It is the little "gremlin" sitting on your shoulder and it is not Jiminy Cricket's voice of conscience. It is an undermining whispering that will bring all of your wondrous ideas and intentions crashing down. For me it was my Grandma Floyd's raspy voice droning, "That's a stupid idea. It'll never work. If it's so great, why hasn't someone thought of it already? What makes you think you could ever do anything like that?" Sadly, we may hear our own voices answering, "Yes, I see what you mean. How did I ever think that would work? How would I ever get the money for that? People will think I'm crazy."

We must, of course look at both the positives and negatives of any idea. If we seriously consider all the pros and cons of the idea and make a rational decision to go ahead with our plans, then the voices can be told exactly where to go when they begin their destruction. They may surface again and again as you work on your project. Tell them, "Thank you very much for your concern, now go away." Continue your project and rejoice when it is completed!

Do you believe that everyone has a purpose here on earth? In order to find that purpose, you must tap in to your creativity. It is never too late to find a purpose. Think of all those who started new businesses later in life! Colonel Harlan Sanders was in his 60s when he founded Kentucky Fried Chicken; Ray Kroc started the franchising of McDonald's when he was 52; Coco Chanel designed her famous woman's suit after coming back from retirement at age 71; Emily Post's *Etiquette* was published when she was 50; John Huston directed James Joyce's *The Dead* at age 80; and John Glenn, officer, astronaut, and senator, literally blasted out of this world at age 77!

Everyone needs a purpose in life. Even if you feel yours is very humble, doesn't it make you feel needed? Contributing to the world as a whole, or to our world in particular, in a meaningful way helps us earn self-respect and the respect of others. A sense of usefulness is essential for satisfaction in life, especially as you grow older. When you have a true purpose or personal mission, you have a sense that you are making a difference in the lives of others.

When you are living your life purposefully, it means every act, task, and situation is worthy of your total attention. You will be going in a direction that is truly your own. Maybe it's time to review your goals. Ask yourself some questions. Are you going in the direction you want? Are you living your life purposefully? Living creatively may ask you to toss aside all your old beliefs and welcome new ones. This can be quite intimidating at first, then rather freeing! Success will come from your ability to enjoy and take advantage of problems. If you are always serious and trying to be reasonable, you are sabotaging your creativity.

## Get in Line

Standing in line has always been a pet peeve of mine. It seems that I always get behind someone who has a problem. On one of those days I saw a young boy standing with his mother obviously feeling the same way. I stared at him. He stared at me. Slowly I opened my mouth and lifted my lips up high showing my teeth. He stared. I pulled my mouth open with my fingers and stuck my fingers in my nostrils. Smiling, he pulled his mouth open with his fingers and stuck his fingers in his nostrils. I pulled my eyes down. He pulled his eyes down. I stuck my tongue out, he stuck his tongue out. I pulled my ears out, he pulled his ears out. We laughed and giggled and made faces at each other, when suddenly it was my turn! That moment in time still lingers in my mind and I chuckle when I think of what that little boy thought of the crazy lady making faces at him.

## Tin Cup or Bust

Isn't it interesting that I used the word "crazy" in the last sentence? It's considered incorrect to act goofy or silly if you are an adult. When I act goofy, it is usually just as a child would act: playfully, laughing, and having fun. Play is at the heart of creativity. It is a good way to stimulate our minds, help us relax, be enthusiastic, even outrageous! Play complements the creative spirit. How sad when people tell us to "grow up." When we are all grown up, we stop growing, and when we stop growing, we die—not in a literal sense, but in a way that sucks all the life out of us.

Paul Hupp, my father, was "creative" his entire life. Many would call him eccentric, and perhaps he was, but I thought he was funny. He was always thinking of new ways to have fun.

Paul lived in Denver, Colorado, for several years, and my sister and I loved to visit him "out West." Colorado was so different from New England. Cowboys, sagebrush, abandoned gold mines, snow-covered rocky mountains, aspens, and no humidity! One morning Paul announced, "I'm going to teach you girls how to read a map." "Sure, Dad, here's a map of Colorado." Opening up the map on the kitchen table he said, "Pick a place you'd like to visit." My sister and I spent the next few minutes checking out different towns and cities in Colorado. We loved the names Boulder, Red Rocks, and Colorado Springs, but the name that jumped out at us was Tin Cup. Visions of an old mining town, tumbleweed, cowboys, sagebrush, and gunfights fueled our enthusiasm.

Paul grabbed the map, his car keys, and a bottle of soda (mixed with his favorite, Southern Comfort) and we jumped in the car. He sat in the back while my sister and I took turns being driver and navigator. "Get out the map, girls, it's Tin Cup or bust!"

Five grueling hours later, we reached Tin Cup. I never knew driving through one state could be so difficult—or dangerous! Our little Chevy Nova, now covered with mud, had forded streams; crossed over rough, rocky dirt roads; avoided a fatal fall into a rock gully four hundred feet below; and found its way through a hidden mountain pass. Exhausted, we surveyed the town. It came complete with a cowboy, tumbleweed, and a "company store." We explored Main Street, and tired from our adventure through the mountains, decided to spend the night.

Twinkling lights up ahead beckoned us into a friendly tavern, and crusty old mountain men bought us a round of drinks, told us chilling stories of black bear and poisonous snakes, and gave us directions to Pete's Cozy Cabins. A sparkling mountain stream gurgled alongside as we snuggled under our flannel blankets, and the wind whispering in the pines coaxed us to sleep. Driving back to Denver the next day was slightly less adventurous, but by gum, we sure knew how to read a map! We never forgot Paul's method of learning how to read a map, and I try to use fun ways to teach my children everything from geography to map reading to opening their minds to their own creative ideas.

### You're Never Too Old to Do Goofy Stuff

Discover and re-experience the child in you. It requires nothing less than your best—playfulness, daydreaming, and foolishness. Things our society discourages. It's okay to daydream. It's okay to be foolish in appropriate situations. It's okay to laugh. A friend of mine attended a parent/teacher conference. The one "problem" her son had, according to the teacher, was that he sometimes daydreamed in class. Who knows what he was thinking? He may have been integrating all that he had learned that day. He may have been contemplating the state of our country and thinking of creative solutions to all the world's problems. Of course, he may have been daydreaming because he was bored, but the teacher could never accept that theory.

Humor is one of the best ways to discover our creativity. Laughing tends to make you look at things in unusual ways because laughter changes your state of mind. Michael Pritchard spoke at the Humor Project's annual conference and said "Laughter is like changing a baby's diaper. It doesn't last, but it sure helps for a while." Sister Anne Bryan Smollin says to get a "laughing buddy." My sister is my laughing buddy. When we are together we laugh and laugh. People look at us and sometimes frown, but most of the time they seem to want to share our laughter. We try to include as many people as we can. Humor fosters the flow of creative solutions because our defenses are down and our mental locks are released. There is a great quote by Ward Cleaver, from the "Leave it to Beaver" show popular in the 1950s: "You're never too old to do goofy stuff." It's true. Be goofy, laugh until you cry, and you'll add 10 years to your life.

Solving a problem creatively may take a little time. Giving time for incubation of ideas gives your subconscious mind a chance to generate ideas. It forces us to suspend judgment, allowing unexpected solutions to come at unexpected times. It is important to write down your ideas. Carry a pen and paper with you at all times; in the car, next to your bed, in your pocketbook. I notice that solutions always seem to come at what I think is the worst possible time, usually just when I am drifting off to sleep. I keep a pen and pad next to my bed for these times, and when I wake up the next morning I am amazed at what I have written. It's great stuff!

Allowing more time to solve a problem gives us greater perception. We can avoid the rigidity that we encounter in the beginning stages. More time

---

### Multitasking

You can still work on the problem with your conscious mind while you are waiting for your subconscious. There are four ways you can do this:

1. Write the problem on different slips of paper and leave them in different areas, on the refrigerator, on the mirror, in your purse or briefcase.

2. Remind yourself of the problem while performing physical activities. Taking a walk, shaving, cleaning the house, or driving to work.

3. State your problem while meditating, daydreaming or resting. Affirm a positive solution. "I now have the perfect answer to this problem."

4. Repeat the problem to yourself once or twice during the day, but then let it go. Try not to become obsessed with it. The idea is to gently remind yourself, but then forget it completely.

results in new and more open observations, and it can lead to interesting or even stunning ideas. Granted, some problems need immediate answers, so you must work on those immediately. But if you have the luxury of the extra time, by all means, use it! Take a deep breath, let it go, and you'll be surprised and excited with the results!

Being creative can help you in all areas of your life. Success comes from having resilience in the face of adversity, and using your creativity can help you adapt to change and unexpected circumstances. Awareness, deep contemplation, and a sense of humor are your best friends in attempting to learn from difficult experiences. Create a life for yourself that you want. Love yourself, be persistent, and never give up. You are a wondrous being and the world is a better place because of you. Living creatively will give you more in your life than you ever dreamed possible. Enjoy life, give back some of what you have been given, and create, create, create!

**How to Be Creative**
- Choose to be creative.
- Look for many solutions.
- Write down all your ideas.
- Define your goals.
- See problems as opportunities.
- Look for the obvious.
- Take risks.
- Dare to be different.
- Be unreasonable.
- Have fun and be foolish.
- Be spontaneous.
- Be in the now.
- Practice divergent thinking.
- Challenge rules and assumptions.
- Delay your decision.
- Be persistent.
- Practice Mind Mapping for any problem.

- Simplify your life.
- Live with joy and abandon.
- Use your imagination.
- Find the child in you.
- Use role models and anti-role models.
- Open your heart.
- Empty your mind.
- Use your gifts.
- Find your life purpose.

Think again about the questions raised at the beginning of the chapter:
- Do you now believe you are a creative thinker?
- Do you know you don't have to be "gifted" to be creative?
- Have you thought of ways to have fun in a "serious" situation?
- Have you used the mind mapping technique?
- Have you tried Leonardo da Vinci's seven principles of creativity?
- Have you started meditating daily?

# 8

# Shelter From the Storm
## Gather a Support System

*When the coffee is hot, and the talk is good, and the feeling is easy,
and the laughter is light, and the memories are many, but the time is too short,
you know you are with a friend.*

—*Ann Landers*

---

If a crisis occurred right now, how ready would you be?

- Do you have a friend you could call in the middle of the night?
- Are you close to your family?
- Is your "domestic foundation" strong?
- Do you have a list of services you would require in an emergency?
- Do you have time for fun?
- Do you have monetary reserves?
- Is it easy for you to ask others for help?
- Do you know what your mother had for breakfast today?

It's no surprise if you answered no to at least a couple of these—and I can probably figure out which ones, too. Not too many people plan for emergencies, so you probably don't have an updated list of important services. After all, isn't that what 911 is for? (Not always.) As for monetary reserves, well, again, few of us plan adequately for emergencies. After all, isn't that what insurance is for? (Again, not always.) You're probably not lacking in friends or family, but you may or may not be close enough to impose when the need arises.

---

## Oops, We Goofed

*You cannot always control circumstances,*
*but you can control your own thoughts.*
—*Charles E. Popplestone*

When my doctor told me I had cancer, I was stunned, horrified. After being assured for a year and a half that the lump growing in my breast was nothing to be concerned about, I was now being told, "Oops, we goofed. It really is cancer. Sorry." After undergoing the biopsy that yielded this horrific news, I was waiting for a ride home from the hospital. Since all my friends were working that day and were unable to pick me up, my doctor told me she would take care of it. A limo driver walked into my room and asked for the patient who needed a ride, and when I stepped into the black limousine, I thought, "I'm a goner. I must have about two weeks left to live. This must be like that last wish thing they give dying cancer patients." Staring out of the tinted windows, feeling as gray and bleak as that cold November day, too frightened to cry, too stunned to think, I was startled by the driver's voice. "Where do I turn?" "Next right, first house on the left." Fumbling for my keys, I thanked the driver and somehow made it into the house.

Chilly air hit my face as I entered, and I turned up the thermostat. The clank and thud of the furnace was a comforting sound. My cat rubbed herself against my legs, thankful to have me back home. My mind was trying hard to function, but it was difficult. I had to stop the fear or it would smother me. I had to think of something, anything except *that other thing*. I called my sister who was waiting for the doctor's report. Shaking from head to toe, I told her, "I have cancer." Her immediate response was, "I'll be right there."

It took her one long, agonizing hour to get to my house, during which time I thought I would lose my mind. Trying to hold on to some form of normalcy, I brewed a cup of tea and left the kettle on warm for my sister's cup when she arrived.

But she was coming. She would be there soon. I could hold on for an hour, knowing that. When she finally arrived, we could only stare at each other with huge, horrified eyes, she asking mundane medical questions, me answering in subdued monotones.

Suddenly the Hupp genes kicked in. "Wait a minute," I said. We both looked at each other with fight and spirit. "We are Hupps. And Hupps don't keel over and die just because someone says we should. We will fight this thing. We will win. We will not let cancer come into our lives and destroy them!"

Thus began my "medical odyssey." With the help of family and friends, the Hupp genes, a team of doctors, nurses, healers, and "angels," I have battled a disease that would be only too happy to see me dead and buried. With a battle cry of hope, a badge of courage and an army of supporters, I have endured nine years of medical crises with a strength I could only have maintained with the help of these heroes in my life: friends who called just to see how I was feeling; drivers with nerves of steel who took me to Boston for treatments; neighbors who brought me home-cooked meals when I was too weak and sick to make dinner; family and friends who supported and carried me (sometimes literally) through crisis after crisis; and doctors, nurses, and technicians who selflessly spent hours nursing me back to life. Thanks to these special people I am alive today.

> *Much of what we call evil can often be converted*
> *into a bracing and tonic good by a simple change of the*
> *sufferer's inner attitude from one of fear to one of fight.*
> —*William James*

## When the Coffee Is Hot

> *Friendship is by its very nature freer of deceit*
> *than any other relationship we can know because it*
> *is the bond least affected by striving for power,*
> *physical pleasure, or material profit, most liberated*
> *from any oath of duty or constancy.*
> —*Francine Du Plessix Gray*

Friends. What memories are brought to mind when you read Ann Landers' and Francine Du Plessix Gray's quotes? Tailgate parties at a ballgame on a lovely spring afternoon? Sharing a cigar with an old friend while watching the races at Saratoga? Helping raise a barn? Bringing your favorite apple pie to a covered dish supper? A barbeque in the backyard? Your memories may include sad times. Hugging a grieving mother at the wake of her son who died in a tragic car accident, opening your home to a friend who lost his in a tornado, helping rebuild a house lost to a fire, being there for your friend whose child committed suicide.

How thankful your friend must have been to have you there! Sometimes all you did was sit and listen, and that's exactly what your friend needed.

How important you were to him at that moment, and he never forgot you for being there.

We all need this kind of support at some time in our lives. Who hasn't lived through a crisis? What did we need when that crisis exploded into our lives, uninvited, unwanted, unexpected? A friend. A spouse, a sister, a mother, a father, a brother, an aunt, an uncle. Someone who could share in our horror, our grief, our pain. Like a solid rock, we needed them to be there for us when our world was crumbling under our feet.

## Survival Gear

Gathering a support system is one of the most important things you can do for yourself. It is necessary. It is your lifeline when you are adrift on an angry, stormy ocean with no life raft or compass to guide you. It is also necessary when seas are calm. Everyone needs someone to bounce things off of, to share everyday happenings with, laugh together at a good joke with, complain about a difficult day to.

I have a friend whose mother calls every week to say hello and to check in, as she lives in another state. One afternoon while I was watching TV with him, the phone rang, and I had the opportunity to listen in to the conversation. It went something like this: "Oh hi Mom, yes, I'm fine. Yes, she's good too. We're just watching a movie. Yes, we went to the diner for breakfast. It was good. I had the French toast and scrambled eggs and Kim had the pancakes." Startled, I realized she had been asking him about our breakfast! Coming from a proper English family, I was never asked what I had eaten for breakfast. No one would ever have thought about it or even cared. (If they had, they would have assumed I'd eaten soft-boiled eggs with toast and marmalade.)

My friend's mother taught me a valuable lesson that day. She taught me a simple way to show someone you care. It might be a silly thing to some people, like my proper English family, but to her it was important to know what her son had eaten for breakfast. How often do we call someone during the day, just to see how they are doing? Have our lives become so busy, so wrapped up in "important" business that we have lost sight of the truly important things in life? Occasionally I call my sister, who is the editor of a busy newspaper. Some days she is in the middle of a meeting and is unable to take the call, but many times my call is like a breath of fresh air. It is the 10-minute break she needs to get her through the next few grueling hours of the day. Sometimes I even ask her what *she* ate for breakfast! We can learn valuable things about our friends and loved ones by asking seemingly mundane, simple questions.

We might learn that they are lactose intolerant and can't eat dairy products, so when we invite them to dinner we know not to serve quiche. We'll know they are scheduled for knee surgery next week and can call that day to offer support and help. In turn, they will know when we are having a rough time and will ask us to join them for coffee. Sharing the little things binds our friendships and holds them together.

**Pets Ahoy!**

> *Most dogs are earnest, which is why most people*
> *like them. You can say any fool thing to a dog,*
> *and the dog will give you this look that says,*
> *"My God, you're RIGHT! I NEVER would have*
> *thought of that!"*

—Dave Barry

Pets are an important part of a support system. Animals may not be able to verbalize, but they get their messages across in other ways. My cat has just jumped up into my lap as I am writing this to remind me to tell you about the ability of a pet to bring unconditional love into your life. It is difficult to describe the look of absolute adoration a dog has for its owner, tail thumping, eyes wide, teeth showing in a big grin. Animals never hold a grudge, never talk back, and always agree with everything we do or say. Isn't that the greatest? They love us unconditionally and can fill a void in our lives that others may not be able to.

My mother always complained about Happy Cat, a mis-named nasty old cat she inherited from my sister. "Cat hair, cat mess, cat food all over the place," she constantly grumbled. Until Happy Cat died of old age, my mother never realized the void the cat had filled all those years. Someone to talk to in the empty space of a big old house, someone to tell her troubles to, someone to complain to when she burned her dinner.

Do you have a pet? It could be a turtle, a bird, an iguana. A beloved pet can be of the utmost help during times of crisis. Dogs and cats are now being brought into nursing homes and senior centers to bring comfort and joy to those who may not have family close by. Seniors who don't want the responsibility of caring for a pet full time can now adopt a pet for the day. A friend of mine suggested "pet sharing." Animals require different amounts of care, so if you decide to get one, take your responsibility seriously.

**Lifelines**

*Well done is better than well said.*
—Benjamin Franklin

We've become a mobile, often rootless people who think nothing of pulling up stakes and moving to completely different towns, cities, and even countries. Sometimes it's to take a new job. Sometimes it's just for a "change of scenery." It can be with family in tow, or all by oneself. It is necessary to create a new support system when we move. If you know when and where you are moving, you can begin right away. Call the local Chamber of Commerce for a list of doctors, dentists, carpenters, movers, houses of worship, telephone companies, insurance agents. Your initial list may change after you have moved, but you will have a good foundation for the first few months you are living there.

Lisbon, Portugal, was the furthest I had ever been from home when I moved there in 1974. Since I didn't speak much Portuguese it was difficult to create a new support system in a strange country. Luckily there was an American already living there who became our contact person in Lisbon, without whose help we would have languished. He had moved to Lisbon seven years earlier and had already established a good support system of his own. He told me to enroll in the Foreign Students Program at the University of Lisbon right away and start learning the language. It was there that I met a large group of American and British students. They helped us find a great apartment, learn the train schedules to the beaches of Estoril, how to make change, get a bus pass, and avoid being taken by unscrupulous taxi drivers. Living in Portugal became an adventure and a lot of fun instead of a period of isolation.

Do you feel lonely? Are you living in a foreign country? Do you feel like you are living in a foreign country? Have you just moved to a new area? Do you feel alone even though you have lived in the same town your whole life? Are you living in an area far away from friends and family?

It is important to create a new support system when you move, but it is just as important to stay connected with your old support system during the transition. Staying connected can be as simple as picking up the phone and calling your mother. (And remember to ask her what she had for breakfast!) In the early 1970s in Lisbon, calling the United States was difficult. International calls had to be done through the operator, the connections weren't very good, and the calls were expensive. Calling my family just to talk was not always possible so I had to find other means of staying connected. Letter writing became a great way of keeping in touch. Today we are fortunate to have excellent long distance calling services country to country and it's easier than ever to stay connected with friends and family all over the world. And now we have e-mail and "instant messaging," too, but there's still nothing like actually talking to a friend or family member.

What a joy for your friend to pick up the phone and hear your voice on the other end of the line. If you are living in another part of the world, your breakfast may be a little different than hers, and I'll bet she would love hearing about it. If you live in a different part of the United States, that could also be true. I grew up in New England where Johnny Cakes are often served. Johnny Cakes, a Rhode Island tradition, began with the earliest American settlers. Native Americans taught the Pilgrims how to grow, grind, and cook corn, and it became a life-sustaining food for them. The original Johnny Cakes were a mixture of water and corn meal and cooked before an open fire and called "Journey Cakes." Easy to pack and keeping well, they were a staple for travelers. It's fun to make Johnny Cakes when I have out-of-town guests, and I enjoy trying biscuits and gravy when I visit "down South." Sharing different traditions brings us all closer together.

If you are feeling lonely or depressed, it's most important for you to connect with friends and family. Lifting your head off the pillow, shutting off the TV, and dialing a phone number may be the most difficult thing you have had to do all day, but you'll get the boost you need to make it through another lonely day in a strange new place. We must find the strength to reach out to others at this time. If no one is home when you call, leave a message and tell them to call you back. Tell them it is important. After all, it *is* important. You need human contact from someone who loves you. (It is also important to see a doctor if your depression persists.)

Now that you have made that first phone call, the rest will be easier. If no one was home the first time, call another friend. Keep trying until you get a human voice on the other end. Make sure you leave a message to call you back. (If you need to use your cell phone while driving, please pull over before you make the call.)

You don't have any friends? Call your co-workers. Call the Welcome Wagon. Call your local clergy. Go to church. Go to town meetings. Volunteer for various community health, politics, or arts groups. Get involved in something that is interesting to you, and you'll meet others who share the same interests. Make the effort. You'll be glad you did.

## What Would the Neighbors Say? (Don't Suffer in Silence)

How many people do you know who won't call someone when they need help or support? Having grown up in a proper English family, all of us going around with our stiff upper lips, we would never have called anyone to tell our troubles to or to ask for help. We were expected to "eat it up, wear it out, make it do, or do without." Unfortunately, one of the things we did without was a good support system. My family had friends, but they were only for the good times. When things were bad, we suffered alone. English culture insisted that we carry on as if everything was just fine, because for heaven's sake, "What would the neighbors say?"

Please don't suffer alone. You don't have to, and it's so much easier to have someone help you carry your load. Life is better when we share both the good and the bad times with people who care about us.

The Internet has provided us with a way to stay in touch with people we know, and we can "chat" with people in other states and even across the world! Yes, be careful out there in cyberspace, but have fun too. The computer cannot take the place of flesh and blood, but it can fill a gap.

### The Swedish Church (Special People)

*All I can say about life is, Oh, God, enjoy it!*

—*Bob Newhart*

Staying spiritually connected is one of the most important aspects of a support system. If you don't believe in organized religion, there's more to spirituality than just a church. Find someone who shares your beliefs and practice them together. There are many different spiritual outlets, and your personal relationship with God, Goddess, a Higher Power, The Universe, Buddha, the Dali Lama, whomever, is important to your happiness and sense of balance and peace. My mean-spirited English grandmother who never attended church used to say, "God can hear my prayers just as well when I'm on my knees in the garden as when I'm in church." She had a point. We can pray or talk to God anywhere, it doesn't have to be in a building. Yet some of the most loving people I have ever met were in a church, when I was a little girl.

I grew up in Rumford, Rhode Island, in an area that boasted at least six churches of different denominations, all within walking distance on a single street. Of the six churches, my favorite was what my grandmother called the "Swedish Church." Our neighbors, the Andersons, were members, as were others with Swedish names; thus the nickname. It was here that I found adults who truly loved children. Instead of scolding us for sampling the cookies before eating the Swedish meatballs at pot-luck suppers, the adults helped us wipe the powdered sugar off our fingers. If we spilled paint on the floor during craft time, they helped us clean it up, and if we forgot our lines for the Pageant, they helped us remember. They loved us unconditionally, and smiled and hugged us everyday—not just on special days like our birthdays. We learned what it meant to "practice what you preach," for these wonderful people truly practiced their faith.

Do you have a spiritual support system? You need one. What is your way of connecting with your spiritual side? Is it a traditional church or temple? A neighbor's living room? An outdoor ceremony on the beach? It doesn't matter as long as it is *something*. Connect with people who share your concept of God in a loving, non-violent way. Let them love and support you. Let them help you when you need it, and be generous about asking for help.

Your soul craves the spiritual. Cultivate this aspect of your life and you will find support and love beyond anything you ever imagined. If the church, temple, or mosque you are attending doesn't feed and nourish your soul, it may be time to find another one. Go "shopping" until you find one that feels right, and connect with your new friends.

**Just Do It!**

*Do or not do. There is no "try."*
—Yoda (The Empire Strikes Back)

Bold, black letters spell "Health, History and Horses" on the sign to the entrance of Saratoga Springs, New York. Tourists in this town get the red carpet treatment, and having spent eight summers here as a tourist, I knew the "tourist" things to do when I moved here permanently. One of my favorites is to take a mineral bath at the Lincoln Bath House and sit in the effervescent waters as the bubbles from the golden mineral waters cling to my skin, soaking out all the toxins and leaving me feeling refreshed and completely relaxed. A Korean doctor visiting Saratoga told me he would be at the baths everyday if he lived here.

The rise of gyms and health clubs is a great thing. Americans are taking better care of themselves and taking the time to exercise, relax, eat better, and even socialize while doing it. There are saunas, steam rooms, whirlpools and lap pools, all for the betterment of our health. Hurrah for good health!

Time, commitment, action. How much time have you committed to your health? Your happiness? Your social life? Yes, it takes a lot of time, work and effort, but the benefits are worth every precious minute. Take time to nurture yourself and your support system. Invite a friend to come with you to jog or go to the health club. Take him or her out for dinner afterwards. Celebrate an accomplishment. Commit to spending a certain amount of time every week taking care of yourself. Make your schedule work around you. This way you can fit in the things you want to do, especially making time for fun.

**Ghosts!**
Halloween is one of my favorite celebrations, and my Halloween party has become an annual tradition. Invitations read, "Come for cider and do-nuts and ghost stories around the campfire." On the night of the party, luminaries light the entrance to my home, and guests are greeted by jack o' lanterns grinning their jagged toothed welcome. Ghoulish shadows dance like skeletons by the glow of the campfire out by the gazebo. Festive black and orange plates hold New York's finest cider doughnuts. After drinking some apple cider, everyone pulls up a chair by the fire and tells their ghostly tales.

Crowding around the fire as it hissed and popped, everyone got quiet as I began my story. I had been living in a rented house in Southeastern New England, close to the ocean. Eerie mists engulfed the house when the fog rolled in, and there were no street-lights on the quiet, deserted dirt road. One night as I was waiting for my friend to arrive, I felt a presence enter the kitchen where I was making dinner. I thought my friend had let himself into the house and I turned around to say hello. No one was there. I swore I felt someone enter the room and searched the house to see if my friend had been playing a trick on me. No one was there. This happened several times and I began to wonder if it could be a ghost. When my landlady told me her story, I believed the presence I had been sensing was indeed the ghost of her late husband, Mason.

Mason and Etti (my landlady) met while she was traveling in Israel. They fell in love, and Mason left his home, his family, and his country to move to the United States to be with Etti, the love of his life. The older couple built the house of their dreams and moved in, living happily for many years until Mason had his first heart attack. He died a year later in the house, and Etti, stricken with grief, closed up the wing of the house containing Mason's clothes, books, and personal effects, and moved out. I believe Mason "lived" in that part of the house.

I felt Mason's presence many times but never felt afraid. I believe he stayed in this world until he and his beloved Etti could leave together. Sometimes our support systems hang around even after they're gone!

Everyone loved my ghost story, but first prize went to my friends who told this one:

Friends of theirs who lived in England bought an old Victorian mansion two hours outside of London. The house boasted many features, including a beautiful staircase leading to the upper rooms. At one point the staircase turned sharply, and there on the landing the owners felt a constant cold spot. No one really thought much of it, assuming it was a draft coming up from the musty old basement. Many years later, while renovating the house, the wall to the staircase had to be replaced, as the wood was deteriorating. The family hoped that by replacing that part of the stairs the constant cold spot would finally be repaired. Horrified screams pierced the air as the wall came down, for dangling there were the remains of a human skeleton!

Everyone at that party enjoyed themselves immensely, anxiously awaiting Part Two of the "Staircase Skeleton" at next year's party. They want answers: who was murdered and hidden behind the wall? Were there any missing persons reports in the town? Is the cold spot gone?

This sort of fun and camaraderie is one important aspect of what we consider a "support system." Support systems are not just there for the bad times.

## Don't Worry, Be Happy

*Most folks are about as happy as*
*they make up their minds to be.*

—*Abraham Lincoln*

My Halloween party guests thoroughly enjoyed themselves that night. Is there some way you could bring more fun and fancy into your life? If you dislike parties, could you go to a movie and then out to dinner? Sometimes we get so caught up in the seriousness of life that we forget to have fun. My grandmother used to get very angry with me because I enjoyed going out as a teenager. "All you ever want to do is have fun," she scolded. Fortunately I didn't listen to her and continued to have fun and, today, still make time every week for entertainment. I take care of my responsibilities first, but always schedule time for a Saratoga Polo game, great jazz at a local jazz club (9 Maple Avenue), or a play at the Spa Little Theater. Summer brings the New York City Ballet and the Philadelphia Orchestra to Saratoga, and I attend many of those performances.

But a good support system requires what I call a "domestic foundation." This consists of people you seldom think of until you need them—and aren't usually the sorts of people you invite to parties or meet for coffee. Do you have an electrician you can call in an emergency? A carpenter, plumber, banker, lawyer, doctor, dentist, massage therapist, senior support service, hospice nurse, insurance agent, veterinarian, librarian, financial planner, handyman, car mechanic, hairdresser, eye doctor? Do you have your emergency telephone numbers on speed dial? Do you know the non-emergency numbers of these support people?

Look at your own domestic foundation. You may know many people you can call for help, and that's great. It is a good idea to have their telephone numbers in a special place so anyone in the house or apartment can find them if necessary. If you have just moved to a new town or city, it's extremely important to implement your new support system and domestic foundation. It's not always wise to wait until an emergency arises and run to the Yellow Pages.

## Water, Water Everywhere

*Not only is there no God,*
*but try to find a plumber on Sunday.*

—*Woody Allen*

When the ink had dried and the real estate agent handed me the keys to my new home in upstate New York, I didn't think I'd be needing the services of a plumber so soon after moving in. Famous last words.... Two weeks later, I awoke to find water gushing from the ceiling onto the beautiful wood floor. The water appeared to be coming from the upstairs bathroom, so I shut off the main water valve. I called a local plumber I found in the Yellow Pages, and when the secretary asked if I had an account with them, I had to say no. "The plumber is out on a call, he'll try to get to you on Monday," was her reply. I had to wait two days for the plumber because I did not have an account with him. If you have just moved to a new town, or if you have been living in the same town for years but do not have an account with a local plumber, establish one. Call the owner of the business, go there and introduce yourself, even send them a check for $10 so that if you have an emergency you will have established an account and get service when you need it, not two days later.

If you have lived in the same town or city for the last 20 years and already have a good domestic foundation, it may be a good time to reassess your list. How is the service you are getting from your insurance agent? Are you happy with your hairdresser? Has your primary care doctor moved to a bigger office on the other side of town?

It may be time to make some changes. Change can be refreshing, but it can also bring feelings of fear. These feelings are normal. Go ahead with the changes anyway, pushing through the fear. The feelings will pass. The elderly may have a difficult time making changes. My mother complains about her primary care doctor but will not change doctors. Change can be difficult and scary, and in some cases, as with my elderly mother, may not be the best thing to do. If you feel comfortable making some changes, by all means do it. You'll wonder what took you so long.

## Support Thyself

A good support system must include a good relationship with yourself. As Eleanor Roosevelt said, "Friendship with oneself, is all important, because without it one cannot be friends with anyone else in the world."

Can you look in the mirror at yourself, naked if you dare, and honestly say, "I love you?" This is one of the most difficult things for most of us to do, and I congratulate you for trying this. I am not talking about a narcissistic or egotistical type of love (which isn't really love at all), but an honest self love.

Listen to your self talk. Most of us have some negative tapes running through our heads, voices from the past, voices from different parts of our lives—arrogant bosses, tired teachers, over-worked parents, jealous siblings, well-meaning friends, autocratic authority figures, intimidating basketball coaches. Not everything they said was positive or for our good. Whose voices are you hearing?

"I'll give you something to cry about!" is the voice my sister hears straight from my Victorian grandmother. Have you ever heard this one? "You'll never amount to anything?" How often have we proved them right? Strangely, my English ancestors thought that by degrading and demoralizing children it would have the opposite effect and make them "turn out right." My family has had to struggle twice as hard to overcome this negative programming. Have you experienced this? It may be difficult, but you can reprogram those negative statements into positive ones that encourage you instead of put you down.

The best way to do this is by replacing the negative statements with positive affirmations. Repeat to yourself, "I am successful. I am a good person. I can do this." Meditating daily can also stop negative banter. Pay attention to your breath and just sit quietly. Try it for five minutes the first time, then increase it to a half hour. If you drift off, or start hearing chatter, focus on your breath, breathe out the thoughts, and begin again. Don't get discouraged if this continues to happen. With practice you will get better. Meditating regularly will be one of the best investments in yourself that you could ever make.

Many of us have hopes and dreams but never achieve them because we don't have anyone to guide us, encourage us, or cheer us on. Those old negative voices block us, slow us down, keep us locked in jobs we don't like, trap us in situations that cause us stress, keep us living in areas that are detrimental to our health. You may want to hire a "life coach" who can help you find the courage to look inside, ask yourself "What do I really want?' and map out a plan to help you get what you want.

### For the Love of Money

Gathering a support system should also include monetary support. Having reserves of money is of utmost importance during a crisis, yet our society focuses more on spending money than saving it. Credit card companies give easy credit, and many people have found themselves in credit card debt. My 18-year old daughter constantly receives "pre-approved" credit card applications, yet she doesn't have a full time job. How is she expected to pay off the bill? We tear them up as soon as we receive them.

After the "Internet boom" of the late 1990s sent technology stocks and the stock market in general soaring, in 2000–2001, the market came crashing down. Many people lost money, yet others who had a more conservative portfolio did not lose as much. If you decide to play the market, it is a good idea to hire a good financial planner. Some people need a more conservative approach to their investment strategy, and a good financial planner can help plan that approach. It is never too late to start saving money. You could begin today by saving just $10 a week. You may never miss it and at the end of one year you'll have saved $520! If you put it in the bank, you'll even earn interest. Somewhat higher interest yields can also be gained by investment services such as money markets and CDs (that's certificate of deposits, although my daughters spend a lot of money on compact discs!).

Should you stay at your present job? Is it time to ask for a raise? Do people owe you money? Should you raise your fees? Do you have a good retirement plan? Do you receive benefits and health insurance? A good monetary support system will give you a strong foundation during a crisis, yet many of us do not have that system in place. Start today to look at your finances, and begin now to implement a plan. Have your financial plan in place before a crisis hits.

Our relationship with money can be as complex as our relationships with people. Most of our beliefs about money we have learned from our families. Have you ever looked at your family's belief system regarding money? It can be very enlightening. What were your family's beliefs about money while you were growing up? Did they judge others more fortunate? Did they look down on others less fortunate? What did your family teach you about saving or spending money? What are your financial goals and dreams? Do you need help with a financial plan? Have you ever been troubled by something regarding money? Financially burned? What have been some financial successes?

"Merry old England" wasn't so merry for my grandparents in the 1920s. Working for wealthy English families, my grandfather as a butler and my grandmother as a cook/nanny, they were disenchanted with low pay and no hope of advancement in their "stations." Aunt Doll, my grandmother's younger sister, had moved to Rhode Island several years earlier, and wanted her sister near her. My grandparents had always dreamed of buying their own home, so they packed their belongings and sailed across the ocean believing in the promise of a new life. Hard work and frugal living paid off. Hearts bursting with pride, they finally bought a cozy bungalow on Barney Street, in the lovely town of Rumford.

Rumford has a fascinating history. It was named after Count Rumford, the Benjamin Franklin of that time. Written out of our history books because he was a spy for England during the American Revolution, he was the first to study diet and vitamins, to invent an effective oven, a smokeless fireplace, and an airtight wood stove. There are few books written about him, but Count Rumford remains a fascinating figure, and it is well worth reading his history.

Anyway, Rumford, Rhode Island, is the original home for Rumford Baking Powder, and the factory still sits in the heart of the town. I loved growing up in Rumford. It was an idyllic place for kids. Parents in Rumford never had to buy their children watches, we could tell time by the factory whistles. Our favorite time of day was when the 5:00 whistle blew, which meant time to go home and watch the Mickey Mouse Club. Even better were the three long blasts at 6:00 A.M. on a snowy morning that announced, "Sleep in, no school today!"

My grandparents lived on Barney Street until they died, living frugally even though they were making more money than they had ever imagined. Their attitude towards money influenced me greatly. Even though they were no longer working for wealthy families, they still looked upon them with some hostility. When I wanted to buy the house of my dreams, I wondered why I was feeling guilty and unworthy of such a house. When I asked myself questions like "What were my family's beliefs about money and others who were more fortunate than us?" I realized unconsciously that I believed my family would judge me harshly for living in such "grandeur." Overcoming that belief was difficult for me but worth it. I bought the house and achieved my dream.

## Life Support

Your "domestic foundation" should include at least some of the following:

| | |
|---|---|
| Doctor | Ambulance |
| Dentist | Hospice |
| Lawyer | Psychologist |
| Handyman | Healer |
| Carpenter | Life Coach |
| Painter | AA |
| Insurance Agent | Pharmacist |
| Senior Support Services | Housekeeper |
| Telephone Company | Travel Agent |
| Internet Provider | Florist |
| Veterinarian | Funeral Home |
| Librarian | Tailor/Seamstress |
| Banker | Hairdresser |
| Financial Planner | Child Care Provider |
| Yoga Instructor | Jeweler |
| Hospital | Pest Control |
| Realtor | Landscaper |
| Laundromat | Lawn Care |
| Dry Cleaners | Optometrist |
| Supermarket/Deli | Cobbler |
| Health Food Store | Acupuncturist |
| Food Co-op | Massage Therapist |
| Car Mechanic | Chiropractor |
| Gas Station | Meditation Center |
| Fire | Bank |
| Police | Coffee Shop |

Once we have looked at old beliefs, it is time to start managing the money we have been given. If this is difficult for you, it may be time to ask for help. Commit to having financial health and a solid financial future. It can be done. It may be difficult to get out of debt and into a program of savings, but you can do it. Ask yourself why you have to drive the BMW instead of the Buick. It is not a bad thing to want the BMW, but if it is causing you financial stress, it may be time to rethink matters. You can begin to save for the BMW, but drive the Buick until you have the reserves to do it the right way.

We can change our beliefs about money, how we handle it, how we save it, how we spend it. Take some time to look at this important area of your life. Your monetary support system can help you attain your dreams and will be a foundation that will help you in times of crisis.

## A Safe Harbor

> *God is our refuge and our strength,*
> *a very present help in trouble.*
>
> —*The Bible*

Finally, in addition to people, a support system should include a place to regroup and feel grounded. Do you have a special place you can go, a haven away from the world, a place you can reconnect with the spiritual and with yourself? Can you carve out a quiet place in your home or office? It doesn't have to be a large space, it could be a special chair in your living room. It doesn't even have to be in your home, just a place where you go to unwind, relax, and renew.

Two old wicker chairs sit in the gazebo behind my house, and it is here that I go to get away from the world. In the summer I sit quietly and listen to the birds and the crickets. In the winter I sit by a crackling fire in the campfire pit behind the gazebo, basking in its warmth. Being close to nature helps me relax and slow down so I can face the rest of the week. You don't have to do this every day, just often enough to keep your stress level down.

Your support system will be unique to you. As you create your support system keep in mind the time, commitment, and action that will be necessary for it to happen. Take the time. Make the commitment. Take action. Use your support system daily to help you with your life, to give you a lift during a hectic day, to be your solid foundation when you are faced with a crisis. By having and using a support system, our lives can be richer, fuller, happier, and easier. Remember, too, that your support system will continue to evolve. One of my coaches once said, "Your address book will constantly be changing." I didn't really understand what she meant until I made out my invitation list for my yearly Halloween party and realized it changed from year to year. Notice how some people come into your life for a little while, then fade out, how others come into your life just at the right moment, and how still others stay forever. Trust your gut feelings when people come in and out of your life. Be aware of their message. Gather your support system and know that when crisis comes into your life, you will be prepared.

---

After reading this chapter, have you begun to improve your support system?

- Have you arranged with a friend to call in the middle of the night if you need to?
- Do you feel closer to your family?
- Have you updated your domestic foundation?
- Do you have emergency numbers on speed dial?
- Have you made more time for fun?
- Have you begun to increase your monetary reserves?
- Have you started asking for help?
- Do you know what your mother had for breakfast?

# Help!

## Actively Seek Help for Those Things
## You Can't Handle Yourself

*God is our refuge and strength, a very present help in struggle.*

*—Psalms 46:1*

Do any of these questions apply to you?

- When you need help, do you ask for it?
- Do you recognize when something is too big for you to handle?
- Do you offer help to others?
- Is it difficult for you to ask for help?
- Do you understand the grieving process?

Sometimes in our push for self-sufficiency, we forget that it's OK to admit when we can't handle something—and that something can be as simple as asking someone to explain a direction in a cooking recipe or help change a flat tire, or something as major as advice and counseling when we have a major health problem. We saw in the last chapter the value of having a support system, but in this chapter we'll start to see the real value of the people in it. Having a support system that you can't turn to for help is like buying an expensive sports car and leaving it in the garage.

**We've Been Bobbed**

> *People must help one another; it is nature's law.*
> —*Jean De La Fontaine*

Waves crashed against the rocks as the full force of Hurricane Bob blew up the coast of Massachusetts and into Westport Harbor. Salty rain slashed downward at an angle, whipping leaves onto the road where they lay like a thick green carpet. The wind roared through the trees, snapping them in half with sharp cracking sounds. Hours later, when the wind quieted down and the torrents of rain slowed, townsfolk peered out their front doors, wondering if it was safe to come out.

The timid left their homes with flashlights, checking for damage. The adventurous ventured down to the beach. The storm surge had broken through the 30-foot-high sand dunes and had washed away much of the beach, creating a sand bar that stretched a hundred yards out to sea.

Many beach homes had been destroyed. Our friend's cottage was found floating down the Westport River, another was on its side, and one that had been tossed across the street displayed a sign that read, "We've been Bobbed." Huge chunks of concrete, once the causeway to the beach, blocked the entrance once used by cars. Sailboats had been tossed like toys onto the streets.

Devastation was everywhere. Power was out for a week. Neighbors pitched in and helped each other. The roar of chainsaws ripped through the air as trees were cleared from the roadway. Those lucky enough to have generators opened their homes to others for a hot shower, a hot meal, and precious freezer storage.

The local supermarket welcomed customers with free coffee and doughnuts during the power outage, and it was here that people gathered to share Hurricane Bob stories.

A sense of camaraderie prevailed. After a week, power was restored, branches and tree limbs had been removed from the road, green gunk that had once been leaves was scraped off windows, and life returned to normal.

**"Help Me If You Can, I'm Feeling Down"**

> *It's the friends you can call up at 4:00 A.M. that matter.*
> —*Marlene Dietrich*

Is it easy for you to ask for help? For many, it's the most difficult thing to do. My family taught me, "I can do it myself."

One of the first times I had to ask for help was during a medical emergency. The infamous "botched biopsy" (when I almost bled to death internally) continued its infamy. The stitches let go, and the wound began to bleed profusely. Horrified at the amount of blood I was losing, I called the doctor. She was quite concerned, and told me to meet her at the hospital. I knew I couldn't drive myself there but honestly didn't think I could ask anyone to help me! I had many close friends, but I had never asked any of them for help. It was a new experience for me, so I called a taxi instead! The taxi driver took pity on me and actually stayed in the waiting room until the doctor had re-stitched the wound, but told me he didn't want me to call him again.

That taught me a lesson. I knew it was time for me to start asking for help. Most people are happy to help someone in need. The greatest outpouring of help I have ever seen came after September 11, when the World Trade Center and part of the Pentagon were destroyed by hijacked commercial aircraft. People didn't even have to ask for it. According to some accounts, ice cream trucks parked by the site gave out everything they had to overheated workers; church tents were raised overnight offering non-denominational services around the clock; homeless people collected money for disaster relief, and children in schools surrounding the Manhattan area drew pictures showing their support of the people of New York City. The city of Saratoga Springs, New York, offered relief workers free hotel and restaurant services. Monetary donations poured into the offices of the Red Cross, and thousands lined up at hospitals to donate blood.

## "See" Sick

*Lots of people want to ride with you in the limo, but what you want is someone who will take the bus with you when the limo breaks down.*
                                                                —*Oprah Winfrey*

After the first phase of my "medical odyssey," I decided to start a new life in Saratoga Springs, New York. The movers had just filled the moving van with my furniture, and I was on the phone with the realtor when I had a call on the other line. It was my oncologist informing me my cancer had come back (my first recurrence). Her words hit me like a ton of bricks. I couldn't see, I couldn't hear. I felt like I was going to pass out. I remember thinking "How can this nightmare be happening to me again?" I told the doctor, "I'm in the middle of moving, I'll call you back."

In a state of shock and disbelief, I arrived in Saratoga. The nightmare was still with me. What was worse was that I had left my entire support system in Massachusetts. I was desperate, lonely, and miserable. My children were worried.

I had to drive myself to a new doctor's office, suffer through a painful bone marrow biopsy, and drive myself home. I cried a lot. I called my sister and my friends from home who supported me as best they could from long distance, but I really needed someone to be with me. Thankfully my treatment consisted of changing my medication with no further chemotherapy that time, but the emotional toll was devastating.

In this age of self-help, self-service, and self-support, we may be lulled into thinking we can do everything by ourselves. We can't. If you have never experienced a crisis before and this is all new to you, you may feel isolated. There are support groups for just about anything nowadays, and most of them are listed in the newspaper, in the phone book, or on the Web. Call them. Join them. Actively seeking help for the things you can't handle is your lifeline during a crisis.

## Don't Be Afraid to Ask

*A pessimist sees the difficulty in every opportunity,*
*an optimist sees the opportunity in every difficulty.*
—*Sir Winston Churchill*

What are some of the reasons we might not ask for help? Many of us might not realize it, but we may simply be too proud. Proud people, according to Webster's Dictionary, usually have "an unreasonably high conception of their own excellence, of their achievements, position, or importance." Sometimes our pride can get in the way of good common sense and stop us from asking for help when we need it. It's like the old cliché about men not wanting to stop and ask for directions. Pride often won't allow them to think that they're lost! But if we step back and look at the situation objectively, we might realize we could really use a little help.

Sometimes we are so deeply involved in the crisis that we can't "see the forest for the trees." When my mother had to be hospitalized for an infected toe, it turned into three months in an assisted-care home because of her uncontrolled diabetes. When she finally returned home, it was a huge transition. My sister was taking care of my mother as well as working full time. My mother was having a hard time adjusting to the "new" routine of being home again, and my sister wasn't sleeping. She called me from Rhode Island one night, beside herself. Because I wasn't so closely involved, I could offer ideas she hadn't thought of. The crisis was resolved quickly. If someone offers some suggestions to a problem you are having, they may be able to "see the forest" and give you sound advice.

Many of us "weren't brought up that way." We learned our responses to life from our families, and many families that I knew in New England were close-knit, tight-lipped, and self-supporting. Asking for help would be considered shameful. This strong spirit of determination is a wonderful asset, yet at times can get in the way.

Are you stoic? Webster's Dictionary defines stoic as "not affected by passion: able completely to repress feeling, manifesting indifference to pleasure or pain." Are you cut off from your own feelings? This could allow you to deny what is happening in your life.

That said, sometimes a dose of "healthy denial" can get us through some rough spots in our lives. When the doctor told me my cancer was back for the third time and had metastasized to my bones, I immediately associated the word "metastasized" with "death." Misinformed people led me to believe that when cancer metastasizes the patient dies. I chose to deny this "fact." I believe part of that denial has helped keep me alive. (The fact is that cancer patients do *not* always die when their cancer metastasizes.)

I did not deny that I had cancer, I chose to be treated with another course of chemotherapy, and took very good care of myself. Yes, I was stoic, and I repressed that little voice that screamed, "You're going to die!" But I got the help I needed. Try this formula: balance stoicism and denial with reality, and get the help you need.

## Keeping Your Boat Afloat

> *It's not the size of the dog in the fight,*
> *it's the size of the fight in the dog.*
>
> —*Mark Twain*

When a crisis hits, our world may feel like a stormy ocean in the grip of a hurricane. Monster waves toss us to and fro. We may feel like we are struggling in deep water simply trying to stay afloat. Our life raft has been smashed to pieces, and we are hanging on for dear life. In other words, we feel like we've been "Bobbed."

What do you need to do to survive? If you need time off from work, take it. If you need to work more, work more. If you need to lie on the couch and watch TV, watch it. You are unique, and the way you cope will be unique to you.

When your life has calmed down and you are feeling better, take stock of your situation. What happened, exactly? Where is your crisis on a level of 1 to 10—1 being the least and 10 being the most? Remember that this is your interpretation, not what "the experts" say. Don't compare your situation to someone else's; this is the time to look at *you*. This is *your* crisis, and you may react to it in a completely different way.

Assess the situation. Look at the whole picture. See what is happening around you. Take a reality check. Is having your head gasket blow up twice in eight months as bad as it seemed two weeks ago? Is it really worse? How are you handling it? Do you need some help?

Do you have a physical problem? Have you had surgery and need help changing dressings or help around the house? Were you fired from your job? Are you sinking into a depression? Have you lost a loved one?

## Using Your Compass to Find Your Way Through Grief

When I was 12 years old, my three-year-old half-brother and nine-year-old step-brother died in a house fire. The tragedy was too big for me to handle at that age. When I was told of their deaths I didn't know how to respond. Counseling was not encouraged for young children in the early 1960s, so I wasn't able to work through the grieving process completely.

It wasn't until years later that I realized the full scope of the tragedy. The thought of my baby brother and step-brother trapped in a burning house was horrific to me, but I could finally grieve in a healthy way.

Today counseling is accepted and encouraged for adults and children. Counseling is beneficial for everyone at some point in their lives. It's helpful to have an objective listener who can help us gain some insights into the problem. A counselor can also help us understand and resolve any feelings that come up. Everyone has their own time frame for dealing with grief. Your feelings may last much longer than someone else's. Usually it takes about a year to fully mourn a loss, but it could be more or less. If the grief becomes chronic and lasts longer than a year or two, you may need some professional help. Take your own time to process your grief, and remember that it's perfectly normal to feel badly for quite some time after a loss. Ask for help if you need it, and talk to family and friends.

One word of caution. Family and friends may be supportive of you and a comfort during a difficult time, but unless they have been trained in grief counseling they may not understand the process. Well-meant advice may not be the best advice. For example, people who tell you only those things that will make you feel better (rather than what the reality of the situation may be) often do you a disservice. It is important to realize that you must handle this in your own way and in your own time. Be patient with well-intentioned advice. Remember that your friends and family love you and want to see you happy again. Even if their advice is wrong for you, the intention behind it is right. Their hearts are in the right place.

You ultimately know what is best for you. Take stock of your situation, be honest, and ask yourself if your behavior is *con*structive or *de*structive. Have you "beaten yourself up" over something? You are special and wonderful, even it you don't feel like it right now. Self–destructive behavior just gets us deeper into the pit of self-pity, and that is not a fun place to be.

## Picking Up the Pieces in the Storm's Aftermath
*A friend should bear his friend's infirmities.*
—*William Shakespeare*

My father never really recovered from the death of his son and stepson and, even after months of counseling, dropped into the depths of despair. He gave up his thriving law practice in Colorado, divorced his wife, packed what little he had left, and drove until he stopped at "the most beautiful place in the world," the little fishing village of Destin, Florida. Here he stopped, rented an apartment, and tried to put back the pieces of his shattered life. He did come back a little, even managed to be happy at times, but he was never the same.

Tragic loss has a way of changing us. We are never the same afterwards. We have lost our innocence. We realize that life can really hurt us, and we are not immune from pain and suffering. Yet we can learn and grow, have more compassion for others, and eventually heal. We will never look at life the same way again, but this can be a good thing. As painful as our crisis can be, it is always an opportunity for growth.

The global pain from the terrorist attacks on the World Trade Center and the Pentagon wounded us deeply, yet incredible acts of kindness and generosity followed. We can give such a gift to others when we have come through a tragedy or loss. There is a light at the end of the tunnel. With help and support from those who love us, we can get beyond the pain and suffering, eventually laugh again, feel joy, and realize that we are not alone. We are all suffering, each in our own way, and we could all use a little help from each other during difficult times. Wouldn't it be great if we could all work together to understand each other, to offer love and encouragement to those who are suffering?

We've been there, now we understand. Let's use this knowledge to bring more joy, peace, and love into the world—helping others when they need it and asking for help when we need it. As Dionne Warwick sang many years ago, "What the world needs now is love, sweet love; It's the only thing that there's much too little of."

It takes courage to offer and accept love. It takes strength to survive a crisis. It takes fortitude to transform a tragedy into something positive. It takes understanding to learn and grow from a disaster. Together we can make it. Together we can get through the worst times. By helping each other, we can be loving, caring beings, capable of doing just about anything.

---

*Courage, like its Latin meaning "heart," is at the center of your being. Continually enlarge your capacity for courage by continually enlarging your heart.*

—*Author Unknown*

---

### Children and Death

When a child experiences death, we should be simple, direct, and honest about it. If the child asks questions, answer as best you can in terms the child will understand. A child should be allowed to express any feelings that come up, including anger and sadness. She should be told it is okay to be angry, and he should be told it is okay to cry. Crying is normal and helps heal the pain.

Accept any emotion the child expresses. There is no right or wrong way to deal with a death, and the child should not be told how to feel. The best way to help a child is to offer warmth and your physical presence. If you are feeling sad as well, share that with the child. If she or he offers you comfort, accept it graciously.

Be patient and understanding during this difficult time. Some children may take longer than others to process the death, and adults should tell them that they can take as long as they need.

Listen carefully to what the child shares with you. Reassure the child that death cannot be "caught" like a cold, and that just because one person died, it doesn't mean anyone else will die soon.

Finally, try to get back to routine as soon as possible, and keep stability in the household. This will help the child feel secure during a frightening and unsure time.

### A Journey Through Grief

**1. Feelings of Grief**—You may experience different feelings while going through the grief process. Some of these may include: anger or guilt, restlessness, a sense of unreality, difficulty sleeping or eating, frequent mood changes, a loss of energy, constant thoughts about the person who died, a need to talk about that person, and difficulty concentrating.

**2. Things That Influence How We Grieve**—We may grieve according to the age of the person who died, our relationship with him or her, the circumstances surrounding the death, our own age in relation to that person, our beliefs, spirituality, and personality.

**3. The Grieving Process**—Grief is a response to loss, and should not be treated as a disease or illness we need to get over. Also, there is no set time to grieve a loss. How soon you learn to live with the death of a loved one depends on your relationship with that person and your ability to adjust to the change in your life.

**4. How to Support Someone Who is Grieving**—Be available to listen. God gave us two ears but only one mouth. Use it wisely. Acknowledge the importance of the death by attending the funeral and sending a card. You could also make a donation in memory of the deceased. It's okay to talk about the person who died, even sharing humorous stories.

**5. Things to Avoid**—Never tell someone that it's time to get back to normal, to start a new life, or it's time to stop grieving. Never tell them things to be grateful for, such as, "At least he won't have to suffer anymore," or, "You had so many good years together." Wait a while to offer these ideas. Don't tell someone to put on a happy face or to hide their grief or to stop feeling their sadness.

**6. What Employers Should Do**—Employers should be sympathetic to their employees. They should be open to discussing time off from work to attend the funeral, and even time away from the office during the first year of the death. The employer can ask about the death, offer condolences, send a card, flowers, or a donation in memory of the employee's loved one. In small companies this might actually happen, but in larger corporations, this may be impossible.

## Facing the Holidays

Facing the holidays after the death of a loved one can be one of the most difficult times for someone grieving. The season can exact an emotional toll on everyone involved. Remember there is no right or wrong way to handle the holidays. Family members may choose to follow old traditions, and others may want to change them. It might help ease the pain to do things a little differently.

Because the grieving experience is emotionally draining, it's important to get plenty of rest during this time. It isn't necessary to do all the things you used to do, such as baking, cleaning, decorating, and entertaining. After all, this year is different from other years.

It's okay if you don't do all the things you used to do. Set limitations and do only the very special or important things. Let the rest go. Share your feelings with one another. Once you have agreed on what you want to do for the holidays, let others know. This might be a time to go away on vacation, or have dinner at a relative's house. Do what feels right for you, but remember that it is healing to be with others who love you. Planning a trip can help keep your mind off painful memories.

Doing things for others may offer the greatest comfort. Perhaps volunteering in your community's soup kitchen can give your loss more meaning by reaching out to others in need. There is no set way to handle the grief and sense of loss during this family oriented time. Work through your grief the best way you can.

---

After reading this chapter, do you have a better sense of when to ask for help?

- When you needed help, did you ask for it?
- If something is too big for you to handle, do you recognize it?
- Have you offered help to someone else?
- Is it easier for you to ask for help?
- Have you talked with a counselor?
- Do you better understand the grieving process?

# **10**

# Blessing of the Fleet
## Find Something to Be Thankful for Every Day

*I've learned that it's those small daily happenings that make life so spectacular.*
*—Andy Rooney*

Think about the following:

- Can you find something to be thankful for every day?
- Can you make problems work for you instead of against you?
- Do you see the glass half-full instead of half-empty?
- Do you feel as though you live in a state of deprivation?
- Do you live your life on an even keel?

If you answered no to any of these questions, you're pretty normal. It sounds kind of corny to always find something to be thankful for every-day, especially in a time when it's fashionable to be cynical. But what purpose does being bitter and cyncial serve? In other words—why should it be so fashionable to be unhappy?

## The Botched Biopsy

*All of them surgeons—they're highway robbers. Why do you think they wear*
*masks when they work on you?*

*—Archie Bunker*

*If you woke up, congratulations! You have another chance!*

*—Quote from the Internet*

"This must be what it feels like to die," I thought as another spasm shook my body. Tiny black dots danced across my eyes. I alternated between teeth chattering and pulling the blankets up to my neck, to kicking them off and sweating buckets, soaking the sheets. My mouth reeked of bile. I felt worse than I had ever felt in my life. "God, am I ever having a bad reaction to that anesthesia."

I stared at the big black clock on the wall across from my bed in the tiny hospital room. It glared back at me…Midnight. "God, please let me sleep," I begged. I watched the second hand merrily sweep around the clock; why did the big hands refuse to budge? Wearily I closed my eyes. When I opened them what seemed like hours later, it was 12:05.

A priest entered the room and asked me if I wanted him to pray with me. "Oh yes!" I answered. Maybe he could get through to God. I seemed to be having a little trouble getting His attention. I wanted the priest to stay, but when he found out I wasn't Catholic, he left in a hurry.

Two agonizing hours later a nurse took my blood pressure. "Do you normally have low blood pressure?" she asked. It was then that I knew. I was "going bad in the night." I had worked in a hospital for a number of years in the Cardiology Department, and this would happen on occasion. A patient would "go bad in the night" and if they made it, they would awaken, wan and weak, surrounded by whirring mounds of blinking, beeping medical equipment. If they didn't, we would see the empty bed in the morning.

Two more nurses swished into the room. I could just barely make out their whispered words, "The surgeon must have nicked an artery during the biopsy, she must be bleeding internally. Call the surgeon and tell her to get here ASAP." In other words, I was going into shock. I was dying.

One emergency surgery, two pints of blood, and three days later, the doctor asked me if I was ready to talk about this. I figured she'd give me the gory details, tell me how to care for the wound, and when to come back to have the stitches removed. Couldn't this wait? I was feeling too weak and dizzy to remember anything. Because of all the blood I had lost, my normally intuitive state of mind was clouded. I hadn't noticed the severity of her words, the way the nurses were tiptoeing around my room, whispering to each other and looking at me with sad eyes. Finally it was time to go home. Finally the doctor and I had time to "talk about this." Finally I heard the words that changed my life forever. I'm glad I was lying down when I heard the words, "You have cancer," so I didn't hurt myself falling prostrate to the floor after hearing them.

"Am I going to die?" Silly question. Of course she would never answer *that* one. It was almost as laughable as when the surgeon told me later "We got it all." The nightmare had begun that day, and although I didn't know it, it was the beginning of my medical odyssey, a journey that has turned out to be the most life changing, fascinating, and horrifying trip of my life.

One botched biopsy, one mastectomy, one bone marrow transplant, two separate years of chemotherapy, two years of Tamoxifen, three recurrences, four major infections, metastases to the bones, lungs, and liver, losing my hair three times, having so many blood transfusions I'm not even me anymore, and nine years later, I have learned to find gratitude for all that has happened to me. Cancer may have been my greatest nightmare, and I agree with Winston Churchill when he said, "If you're going through hell, keep going." I have been to hell, lived my worst nightmare, but my experience with cancer has also been my greatest gift. Being able to get to the point of being thankful for all I have endured has been a process, one I wish to share with you.

### Finding the Pearl in the Oyster

*If you don't like the way life looks, try changing the way you look at life.*
—Lisa O. Englehardt

In a world filled with sickness, death, violent crime, terrorist attacks, high school shootings, disappointments, crises, and constant and rapid change, it may be difficult for many of us to grasp the concept of gratitude. How can we be thankful when bad things happen to us? The simple answer is, we can't. There was no way I was thankful for the hell I went through. If I could have avoided any part of it I would have. But what would I have learned? Have we ever learned a life lesson when our lives were running smoothly and easily?

Being thankful helps us learn to acknowledge and appreciate what we have now, at the present moment. Once we face our fears of the future and let go of the "what ifs," we can practice acceptance. We can accept what we have been given, learn the lesson, grow from the experience, and eventually be thankful.

Once we can learn and accept the idea of being thankful, we can turn the disappointment, injustices, and unfairness around. We can make these problems work *for* us. Just as there will always be upsetting and difficult situations in our lives, there will always be the positive, successful, and joyful side of life. They coexist simultaneously. It is our decision which side we choose.

Choosing gratitude can change what we already have into enough and help us appreciate what we have instead of always wanting more. It can change a simple family dinner into a joyous feast, a sterile house into a warm, cozy home, and a dull life to one full of enthusiasm. It can turn a stranger into a friend, a problem into a challenge, and a feeling of despair into one of hope.

Finding something to be thankful for every day unlocks the fullness of life and makes things feel all right. When you are faced with what seems like a failure, you can turn it around and and into a success. A "cabin fever" trip to Florida deteriorated into disaster when two feet of snow fell the day my daughters and I were supposed to fly out of Albany, New York to Marco Island, Florida. We had been sitting on the plane for two hours waiting to be de-iced when the flight attendant announced that instead of taking off for warmer weather, we would be taxiing back to the terminal to deplane. Our flight had been cancelled along with every other flight south. We were lucky to get out of Albany two days later. Instead of flying to the west coast near Marco Island, we had to fly into West Palm Beach, the complete opposite side of the state. "Let's turn this into a positive, " I suggested to two very ticked off teenagers. I called my brother and sister-in-law who live north of West Palm Beach and arranged to meet them. We spent our first night in Florida with family, and basked in the love and warmth we received from them. (And got to eat delicious home-cooked food!) My oldest daughter intended to apply to the music school at the University of Miami, so we drove to Coral Gables the next day to tour the campus. Later that afternoon we arrived at Marco Island, and although our trip was cut short, we enjoyed the time we had. What could have been a "negative" situation turned into a wonderful opportunity. Can you think of something that may be happening in your life that you could turn around and use to your advantage?

### Live Life as a Moon Tide Rather than as an Ebb Tide
*If it ain't broke, fix it until it is.*

—*Internet Joke*

When we allow ourselves to be thankful for every thing that comes into our lives—whether we perceive it as either good or bad—our past makes sense, the present is filled with peace, and we can create a vision for tomorrow that we know is just right for us. We may have to work on the past, and this can be difficult. It involves uncovering old wounds, allowing the old feelings to surface, cleaning those festering, infected feelings, and healing the area. It takes a lot of courage to do this.

When I was growing up, I craved "normal" parents. Being the only kids in the neighborhood whose parents were divorced, my sister and I were "different." As a child, I wept over my father's apparent indifference to my existence, and the "loss" of my mother because she had to work to support us. My friends' mothers all stayed home. I used to say, "Everyone wants the perfect parents, but nobody ever gets them." I felt resentful of my imperfect parents who I felt had been solely responsible for my difficult childhood. I constantly cried, "Poor me. Poor me." If only I'd had better parents I would have been more successful, better adapted, happier, chosen a better course for my life. I loved to throw "pity parties" for myself.

During my "awakening," I did a lot of inner work, investigating my past and healing old wounds. I looked back at my parents and listed their strengths and weaknesses and how they contributed to who I am today. I realized that without these exact parents and all they came with, I would not be me. It was a revelation and allowed me to forgive them for all the injustices I felt I had received. It freed me to actually thank them for all the pain and suffering I felt, because I had grown in areas I never would have without those experiences. Forgiving them also allowed me to see their goodness and strengths, unfettered by ill feelings.

Once I had accepted the reality of my past, forgiven those who had hurt me, grieved my imperfect childhood, and accepted it all, I was healed. I realized that all my wonderful qualities were inherited from my parents and grandparents. I rejoiced in the idea that I really did have the perfect parents. Hurrah! Can you look back at your probably less than perfect childhood and discover that you too had the perfect parents?

One of the ways we cut ourselves off from thankfulness and a fuller life is by living in a state of deprivation. If we are constantly thinking, "Everyone else has more than me, there will never be enough," we miss the opportunity to live in abundance. *Anyone* can live a more abundant life, regardless of their circumstances. The movie *The Gleaners and I,* a French documentary by Dr. Agnes Varda, shows how some people have lived "in abundance" from discarded food and "trash." To *glean* means "to gather grain left behind by reapers." Dr. Varda's documentary included people who gleaned food from farmer's markets, "imperfect" potatoes dumped in a field and those who picked up items left on the street for the trash man. One man she interviewed told her he had been eating discarded restaurant food for ten years and hadn't been sick once. Two others proudly showed off their home furnished by "junk" and felt they were living an abundant life.

My mean old Grandma Floyd ensconced the belief of deprivation in me. I still hear the words, "We can't afford that!" which was her standard reply to any question involving money. I used to say the same thing before I even checked out how much something cost!

Living in a constant state of deprivation causes us to feel resentful and jealous of people who seem to have more than we do. There was a woman who lived across the street from my family who never had to work. Her father had left her enough money in a trust that kept her quite comfortable. My grandmother called her "The Duchess," and every time she saw her, would make snide remarks. It appeared that "The Duchess" had more than we did, but she had no other family and lived by herself. Could she have been jealous of our family because she never had children?

In my family we hoarded what we had and we didn't really enjoy things much because there was a constant nagging feeling that once it was gone we would never get any more. This type of thinking created a "Why bother?" mindset. Mean old Grandma Floyd's philosophy created a lack luster, stingy, callous way of living, and made Ebenezer Scrooge look like Santa Claus.

Other things that take us away from feeling thankful are overeating and then beating ourselves up for not having the "perfect" body; comparing ourselves to others and always coming up short; competing with people and wasting valuable energy trying to do better; dwelling on painful memories that cause us to feel bad; and imagining future painful scenes that may never happen. We must stop all that. We are inherently good and are all doing the best we can with what we have.

## Expressions of Gratitude

> *Laugh and the whole world laughs with you,*
> *cry and...you have to blow your nose.*
> —*First grader finishing a well-known proverb*

What does gratitude feel like? Can we force ourselves to feel this? Of course not. It's like forcing yourself to get to sleep. Gratitude is simply another way of perceiving the world. We must be diligent in developing thankfulness, for it

---

### Attitude

"The longer I live, the more I realize the impact of attitude on life. Attitude, to me, is more important than facts.

"It is more important than the past, than education, than money, than circumstances, than failures, than successes, than what other people think or say or do. It is more important than appearance, giftedness, or skill. It will make or break a company...a church...a home.

"The remarkable thing is we have a choice every day regarding the attitude we will embrace for that day. We cannot change our past...we cannot change the fact that people will act in a certain way. We cannot change the inevitable. The only thing we can do is play on the one string we have, and that is our attitude.

"I am convinced that life is 10% what happens to me and ninety per cent how I react to it. And so it is with you....

"We are in charge of our attitudes."

*—Charles Swindoll*

---

is not a concept our culture encourages, develops, or teaches us. Thankfulness can feel like a pleasant, tender feeling of warmth, sympathy, or obligation toward someone who has treated you kindly. Thankfulness can also be a sudden rush of feeling towards a Supreme Being, nature, the Universe, or to a situation that delights you.

Thankfulness can be private or public, a whispered "Thank you" or a full blown "Hurrah!" We can express it any way we choose. We must open up our hearts to let the feelings in. It can only happen in the here and now, as it is almost impossible to be thankful for something that is just a possibility. Sometimes we try to force ourselves to feel thankful with a "Things could be worse attitude." When I was in the hospital with the botched biopsy, I tried to feel grateful for something about the whole experience. I remember thinking, "I'm thankful I didn't go home from the hospital like I was supposed to. I'm thankful the nurse discovered the bleeding artery before it was too late. I'm glad it wasn't New Year's Eve and the surgeon didn't stumble into the operating room with liquor on her breath." These are examples of "negative" thankfulness and don't really work. We feel more relief than anything else.

What are some positive expressions of gratitude? Self-nurturance is important because, in effect, we are giving ourselves unconditional love. Every morning, wouldn't it be great if we looked in the mirror and could honestly say "I'm so thankful for this imperfect body. Thank you for my crazy family, and my difficult life. Thank you for letting me be me." Try this tomorrow morning when you get up. Ask yourself, "What can I do for myself today? What will make me feel good? What do I need to do to take care of myself? Who can give me encouragement and support?" Then say, "If I make a mistake I will not beat myself up. I will allow myself to be human."

We must be careful not to become narcissistic. The important thing to remember is that when we take care of ourselves, when our needs are met and we accept and love ourselves unconditionally, we will be able to and will want to do the same for others. If we become totally focused on ourselves to the exclusion of others, it is not true self love.

A second expression of gratitude is self-discipline. Sometimes we need to wait for something; the results of a CT scan, our son or daughter to arrive on a late evening flight, the results of an exam we have taken. When we are in a place of waiting, wanting that thing in the future to happen, it is most important to stay in the moment. By staying in the moment you will be able to pace yourself, stay calm, and find the patience to wait.

Disciplining ourselves is not easy. We are tested daily. At Easter time I am always tempted by the Cadbury chocolate creme eggs in their brightly colored foil wrappers. I must admit that my self-discipline weakens and I succumb to my sweet tooth. My pledge is that I will buy only one (at a time). I will limit myself to a certain number until Easter. Then I will stop. I will not beat myself up and I will savor every bite. Self-discipline will begin again tomorrow!

## Taking Care of Ourselves
*Many people die at 25, and aren't buried until they are 75.*
—*Benjamin Franklin*

Self-care is another expression of gratitude. Once we begin to be responsible for ourselves, our actions, our thoughts, our re-actions, we can open ourselves to the goodness and richness of life. Many of us may not realize the responsibilities that come with being human! We are responsible for leading our own lives in a positive, healthy way, and attending to our needs so that we can set and achieve goals. It is our responsibility to enjoy life as best we can with what we have and to find pleasure in daily activities instead of complaining and finding fault. We are responsible for whom we choose to love and how we choose to express this love and how we allow others to treat us. If we find ourselves in a space we are not happy with, we must ask ourselves, "How did I get here?" and "What will it take to get me to a better place?" Then we must take action to get ourselves there.

When we take care of ourselves, we must practice mutual self-respect by allowing others to live their lives as they choose and not allowing them to interfere with the way we have chosen to live. Many control issues will come up when we do this. I recently met a woman who loves to worry about her children. If they are away, she imagines the most horrific things happening to them, and when they are home, tries to keep them there. She doesn't realize it, but unconsciously she feels that by worrying about them, she will have some control over them. The truth is that we have no control over other people's lives, although we may try to gain control. Most of us have the need to control things in our lives so that we can keep order. This is normal and human. It is when we try to exert control over others to the extent of taking over their lives and not letting them make their own choices, that it becomes unhealthy.

As for ourselves, we must know what we need in order to get our needs met, and we should never punish ourselves for having those needs. Our needs may be different from day to day, moment to moment. As we grow and take better care of day to day obligations, we can forgive ourselves when we make mistakes, congratulate ourselves when we have succeeded, and say, "Well done!" It is at this point that we can develop gratitude for our efforts. There are other times when we aren't up to doing our best, or we just don't feel like it. That's okay too. We will always have ups and downs, feelings, thoughts, fears, and vulnerabilities as we stumble through life. Be easy on yourself when you make mistakes or are having a bad day. You are entitled to it.

It is important to make decisions that enhance our self-esteem and to be grateful for the choices that come our way every day. We can look back at all the good decisions we have made as well as appreciate all the gifts and talents we've been given. Taking care of ourselves includes trusting our decisions, asserting ourselves when necessary, respecting ourselves and the decisions we've made, honoring and being true to ourselves, and being thankful for our presence here on earth.

An essential part of being able to feel thankful is accepting reality. We must face and come to terms with what is actually happening, what is real at this particular moment. It is at this point that we will find the peace in the situation and, frequently, a turning point for change.

This is much easier said than done. It is up to us to either accept or reject the reality of our own particular circumstances. This may include: who we are, where we live, who we live with or without, where we work, our method of transportation, how much money we have, what our responsibilities are, what we do for fun, and any problems that we may be having.

Most people strive to live their lives on an even keel. They seek a level of comfort that works for them and try to live within that comfort zone. When all hell breaks loose and a "bad" thing happens, that balance gets disrupted. Things are changing and becoming different. We may be experiencing loss, and our present circumstances are no longer as comfortable as they were. Something in our life has been altered, and we have a new situation to accept. Our response to the event depends on the severity of the change or loss. We could go into denial, resist the change, fantasize that things will stay the same, or wish that the problem be solved quickly. We want to feel comfortable again, feel the status quo, and know what to expect. We may not feel peaceful with the reality we are now facing; it feels awkward and we are out of our comfort zone. We may feel as though we have temporarily lost our balance.

## Turning the Tides (Keeping Balance During Change)

Portugal's Revolution of 1974 threw the entire country off balance. I was living there at the time, and I saw the Portuguese people react quite admirably. After living under a dictatorship for many years, they suddenly had to adjust to a new form of government. Not knowing what to expect, they took care of the things they could. Family safety and health came first, and next was finding employment during a time of drastic change. It took only a few months for the Portuguese to find a way to exist under an entirely new set of laws, and within one year, the country was operating almost back to normal. They accepted the reality of their new situation, were flexible enough to make some changes, and by keeping as normal a life as they could, survived in new circumstances.

Accepting reality does *not* mean adapting to an unacceptable situation, resignation to a less than ideal life, or tolerating any kind of abuse. It means simply acknowledging and accepting our circumstances as they really are at this precise moment. Once we have done that, we can find the peace and the ability to evaluate the circumstances, make any changes that are necessary and appropriate, solve the problem at hand, and find the power and the strength to do what we have to do. The Navajo have a concept called *hozho* meaning roughly, "If I can't change it, I get in harmony with it."

A friend of mine was living a life she called the "golden handcuffs." She had a beautiful home, a brand new car, and the job she had always wanted. Her husband was successful and paid all the bills. All she had to do was get up in the morning, go to work, and let him do the rest. The marriage worked for awhile, but eventually she realized her husband had been verbally abusive for most of the time they had been together. It was difficult to leave him because she had everything else in her life that she wanted. She finally realized that she was using work as an excuse to avoid coming home at a decent hour. She was really avoiding her husband. It took great strength and effort for her to leave the marriage, as he insisted he was not at fault for their problems. She did not blame him, but knew this was not acceptable for her emotionally.

### Poor Me (Self-Victimization)

> *Instead of waiting for someone to bring you flowers,*
> *why not gather your own bouquet.*
> —*Quote from a poster in a physical therapist's office.*

Some people live as victims. A victim thinks, "This is not the way things should be. I deserve better. Why do bad things always happen to me?" The problem with the victim role is that the problems never go away. The victim constantly blames everyone else for anything that is not right in their lives. When playing a victim role, you lose power and feel you are not in control of your situation. All the problems coming your way are always somebody else's fault. Some people choose to live this way because they may get their needs met by others who love to rescue. This may work for awhile, but the consequence is that the victim never gets beyond the present situation and perpetuates it. They can never be happy or find anything to be thankful for, and may feel depressed.

The way out of this type of thinking is that you can't always control what happens to you, but you can control your response to it. You may think that the Universe/God is random, cruel, or judgmental, but I believe God is wise and compassionate, not wishing "bad" things to happen to us. Even when we feel pain, and our pain is deep, there is always a lesson to learn if we can get to the point of accepting the reality we have been given. Instead of perceiving the world as right or wrong, good or bad, why not see it instead as an opportunity for growth?

You can also use your knowledge about your particular problem to help others. Christine A. Adams said, "Helping others benefits them, makes you appreciate your own gifts, and improves your mood."

Helping others does not erase your own pain. Your feelings of pain are valid and are exquisitely yours. Don't avoid the pain. Feel it and use it as an avenue to spiritual growth. Once you can surrender the anger, pain, bitterness, and feelings of resentment, there is room in your heart for love. And love is the other side of gratitude.

### Accepting Acceptance

Acceptance is the ultimate paradox because we cannot change who we are until we know and accept who we are. When we do this, we can let go of the need to resist ourselves and our environment and are free to feel contentment and to find thankfulness in our hearts.

Acceptance is not a one time thing. It is not forever. It is for today, for the present situation. Wouldn't it be great if we only had this one problem to work through? Unfortunately life does not work that way, and it seems like once we get one thing handled, something else comes up. That is why it is so important to have good coping skills that are well honed. It is so much easier to handle problems if we realize they come along with life. We will never be able to avoid them. If we try to avoid them using alcohol, drugs, or other addictive behavior, it only creates more problems. Accepting what happens to us and resolving those problems is the first step to feeling gratitude for all the problems that come our way.

Acceptance can be one of the most difficult things we ever have to do. There is a five step process outlined by Elizabeth Kubler Ross, a medical doctor, psychiatrist, and internationally renowned thanatologist who has written several books on death and dying. She was one of the pioneers who summarized coping mechanisms used at the time of a terminal illness. Her summary has been called the grieving process as well as the forgiveness process, the healing process and even "the way God works with us."

It is awkward and painful to go through, yet is necessary for us to get beyond our pain. While we are going through this process, we may feel as though we are falling apart. We may feel confused, lonely, isolated, out of control, and may fear we are losing our minds. This may be a time to gather friends, call a professional, or retreat into yourself. Depending on the nature and scope of the loss, it may take a few days or a lifetime to work through.

Be gentle with yourself during this time. Working through the healing process can deplete your energy and throw you off balance for awhile. It is normal. Don't feel as though you are the only person this has ever happened to or that you are going insane.

## The Healing/Grieving Process

*With healing, bones become stronger in the places that were broken. The same is true of broken hearts.*

—*Jack Wintz*

**Step One: Denial and Isolation**—The first step in the healing process is usually denial. We may feel shock, numbness, panic, or a general refusal to accept the reality of the situation. We may pretend it is not happening. Our minds may trick us into thinking things are back to normal, or we may fantasize that it never happened. We may experience severe anxiety and fear. Reactions may be:

- Refusing to believe reality: "No, this isn't really happening, it just can't be!"

- Denying and minimizing the importance of the loss: "It doesn't bother me, it's no big deal."

- Denying feelings about the loss: "I don't care about this."

- Mental avoidance about the loss: sleeping too much, keeping too busy, indulging in compulsive behavior, obsessing.

- May feel detached, like we are "not really here."

- Emotional responses may be dull, flat, non-existent, or inappropriate.

Denial can help us through the initial phase of the process. It can soften the blow of the situation and protect us from our pain for a short time. It is a natural reaction to pain, loss, or change. Denial can ward off the "sucker punches" we may encounter until we can gather our support system and our coping resources. We will move on when the time is appropriate.

**Step Two: Anger**—We may blame others, ourselves, or God for the loss or change. Our anger may range from feeling somewhat angry to full blown rage. It may build up over time and then regress, or we may steep in it for awhile. It can turn to bitterness and resentment. We must be careful at this stage to avoid confrontations and making accusations. The best way to handle the anger is to find healthy outlets for it, such as pounding a pillow, finding a safe place to let out a scream, or using physical exercise to get out some of the anger.

**Step Three: Bargaining**—We may try to make a deal with God, with life, with ourselves, or another person. At this stage we are not trying to postpone the inevitable, we are trying to stop it from actually happening.

**Step Four: Depression**—It is here that we actually acknowledge the loss or change and can start to cry. We may feel very sad and depressed. Once we begin to cry, we can begin to let go. We feel the grief, we are in true mourning, and it is here we feel the loss with all its mighty force. It is important that this step be worked through completely.

**Step Five: Acceptance**—We finally are at peace with what is. We can be free! We can leave, we can stay, we can begin to plan and make decisions. We have accepted our loss. It has become an acceptable part of our lives at present, in the moment, and we have adjusted to the new situation. We are once again comfortable with our lives as they are right now. We are back in our comfort zone.

**Calm Seas, Clear Sailing**
*Have a purpose in life, and having it throw into your work such strength of mind and muscle as God has given you.*
—*Thomas Carlyle*

We feel different once we have done the entire healing process. We feel we have changed and grown. We're not sure why or how, but the feeling is there. We can finally stop running from the pain, trying to control the past, hiding from the future, and avoiding the inevitable. We can move forward!

It is now that we can make goals. Goals are gratitude in action. They give us the chance to begin again with a fresh outlook and with direction and purpose. Goals generate enthusiasm and interest in living life again. There are powerful forces at work behind the scenes: psychological, spiritual, and emotional. They are all working together to move us beyond the pain and suffering of our loss and forward to a more evolved being. We can finally feel gratitude and feel thankful and happy again.

### Some Things I Feel Grateful For

- My wonderful children and family
- My beautiful home and enough food to eat
- All those involved in helping cancer patients
- My continued good health
- My doctors, nurses, support people
- All the musicians, artists, writers, and creative people in my life
- Being able to use all the gifts God has given me
- Being able to see, hear, taste, touch, and smell all that nature has to offer
- Being able to laugh at life and myself
- All my wonderful friends and those who support me on my journey through life

Please list at least 10 things you are grateful for.

After reading this chapter:
- Have you been able to find something to be thankful for every day?
- Have you been able to make problems work for you instead of against you?
- Do you now see the glass half-full instead of half-empty?
- Have you changed from living in a state of deprivation to a state of abundance?
- Are you living your life on a more even keel?

### 10 Commandments for Keeping Ship-Shape

*—Author Unknown*

1. Don't miss the boat.
2. Remember that we are all in the same boat.
3. Plan ahead. It wasn't raining when Noah built the Ark.
4. Stay fit. When you're 600 years old, someone may ask you to do something really big.
5. Don't listen to critics; just get on with the job that needs to be done.
6. Build your future on high ground.
7. For safety's sake, travel in pairs.
8. Speed isn't always an advantage. The snails were on board with the cheetahs.
9. When you're stressed, float a while.
10. No matter the storm, when you are with God, there is always a rainbow waiting.

# Index

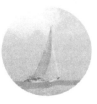

# About the Author

Kim Hupp was born in Denver, Colorado, but spent her childhood in Rumford, Rhode Island. She received a Bachelor of Science degree from the University of Rhode Island, and taught English as a Second Language at the American Language Institute in Lisbon, Portugal. She studied Portuguese language and culture at the University of Lisbon, and business accounting at Bristol Community College in Massachusetts.

Kim was diagnosed with Stage III Infiltrating Lobular Carcinoma in December, 1993. She had a mastectomy followed by chemotherapy, radiation, and a bone marrow transplant. A year later she had reconstructive surgery. She was cancer-free for two years until the cancer returned, and was found in the bone marrow. Oral medication put her back into remission.

One year after that the cancer returned again, this time in her bones. Once again, oral medication worked. Six months later the cancer had traveled to her lungs, and was spreading into more of her bones. She started chemotherapy again, every week for 15 months. This chemotherapy slowed the growth of the cancer, but it eventually metastasized to her liver. She began an oral form of chemotherapy, which lowered her tumor markers and is keeping the cancer stable.

Kim is a shining example of how, with courage and determination, anyone can learn to live not only with cancer, but any sort of persistent crisis. Instead of looking at grim statistics, she chose to focus her attention on living, filling her days with as much fun, laughter, and love that life can give her. She spreads enthusiasm and inspiration wherever her paths take her, and is a sought-after speaker for cancer groups. She teaches seminars and gives workshops, and participants always leave armed with tools to use for not only the "big ones" of life, but for all the little crises we encounter in our daily lives.

Presently living in Saratoga Springs, New York with her two daughters, Kim is already working on her second book. She is a member of the International Women's Writing Guild, and volunteers at various organizations.

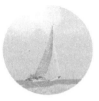

# Resources

The following are some groups, organizations, or shops you may want to add to your domestic foundation list (see chapter 8). Some can provide help with everyday micro-crises, while some are designed to help when the "big one" hits.

**Diet/Nutrition**
Four Seasons Natural Foods Store & Café
33 Phila Street
Saratoga Springs, NY 12866
(518) 584-4670

Saratoga's center for natural foods since 1988. Delicious natural foods cuisine.

Healthy Nation Discount Natural Market
110 Milton Avenue/Rt. 50
Ballston Spa, NY 12020
(518) 885-9999

"Eat better, last longer." Advice and help for choosing healthy foods and supplements.

**Health and Fitness**
The Crystal Spa
120 South Broadway
Saratoga Springs, NY 12866
(518) 584- 2556

Private mineral baths, facials, reflexology, manicures, massages, pedicures, herbal wraps.

Haven Animal Hospital
2686 Rt. 9
Malta, NY 12020
(518) 583-7865

Because pets get sick, too!

Health Journeys
Image Paths, Inc.
891 Moe Drive, Suite C
Akron, Ohio 44310
(800) 800-8661
(330) 633-3831
Fax: (330) 633-3778
info@healthjourneys.com
www.healthjourneys.com

Guided imagery tapes and CDs for almost anything; health conferences, and education.

Lincoln Mineral Baths
Saratoga Spa State Park, South Broadway Entrance
Saratoga Springs, NY 12866
(518) 583-2880

Healing mineral baths and massage, aromatherapy, reflexology, body wraps, facials.

Mana's Yoga Studio
2 Franklin Square
Saratoga Springs, NY 12866
(518) 581-0790  Mana
(518) 893-2350  Nora

A place of beauty and quiet. Classes at many levels, morning, noon, and night.

Menges & Curtis
472 Broadway
Saratoga Springs, NY 12866
(518) 584-2046

Old fashioned style pharmacy with modern care.

Reiki Room
487 Broadway
Saratoga Springs, NY 12866
(518) 580-8988
www.reikiroom.org

A center for relaxation, pain management, stress relief, energy therapy for body, mind, and spirit.

Saratoga Wellness Alliance
376 Broadway
Saratoga Springs, NY 12866
(518) 583-0339

Provides massage therapy, yoga, tai chi, meditation, acupuncture, and more.

YMCA Downtown Facility
262 Broadway
Saratoga Springs, NY 12866
(518) 583-9622

Local fitness center.

**Spirituality**
Malta Ridge United Methodist Church
792 Malta Avenue Extension
Malta, NY 12020
(518) 581-0210
revdebp@yahoo.com

Debbie Peacock, Pastor

**Automotive**
AAA Northway
Auto & Travel
26 West Avenue
Saratoga Springs, NY 12866
(518) 587-8449

24-hour roadside assistance, travel itineraries, and other cures for automotive ills.

**For Fun**
Off-Broadway Theatre & Grill
86 Congress Plaza
Saratoga Springs, NY 12866
(518) 587-3456

The ultimate dinner and a movie!

Saratoga Film Forum
320 Broadway
Saratoga Springs, NY 12866
(518) 584-FILM
www.saratogafilmforum.org

Saratoga's alternative cinema.

**Health/Crisis Organizations**
AIDS Council of Northeastern New York
229 Washington Street

Saratoga Springs, NY 12866
(518) 587-8052

Resources and support for HIV positive and people with AIDS.

Alcoholics Anonymous
Saratoga Springs, NY
(518) 587-0407

Support for people with alcohol abuse problems.

American Cancer Society
200 Osborne Road
Loudonville, NY 12211
(518) 438-7841
(800) ACS-2345 (24-hour information, with oncology nurse on duty)
380A Glen Street, Glens Falls, NY 12801
(518) 792-5358
www.cancer.org

ACS programs include Reach for Recovery; Look Good, Feel better; Road to Recovery; The Loan Closet; Wig Bank; and Image Center. Speakers Bureau: Composed of leaders in the medical field and breast cancer survivors; available in all counties.

Capital Region Action Against Breast Cancer (CRAAB!)
Women's Building
79 Central Avenue
Albany, NY 12206
(518) 462-4472
Fax: (518) 462-0776
www.CRAAB.org

This is a grassroots advocacy group of breast cancer survivors, their family and friends who have open meetings the fourth Tuesday of each month for program development, business planning, and personal support. CRAAB'S "Conversations About Breast Cancer" educational series has monthly meetings to discuss books and scientific journal articles on a wide range of topics with speakers, panel discussions, and healing workshops. CRAAB! organizes annual Advocacy Days at the NY State Capital with other members of the New York State Breast Cancer Network. CRAAB! promotes research and awareness of the environmental links to breast cancer, and works with local groups to increase education and outreach to medically underserved communities.

The Humor Project, Inc.
480 Broadway, Suite 210
Saratoga Springs, NY 12866-4242
www.HumorProject.com <http://www.humorproject.com/>
(518) 587-8770
Fax: (800) 600-4242

Since 1977, The Humor Project, Inc. has been the leading organization in the world focusing on the positive power of humor and creativity. They have a lot of fun along the way, but what they do is not for fun: their goal is to provide services, programs, and resources that make appositive difference in the lives of individuals and organizations...to help you get more smileage out of your life and work!

Learning-filled, laughter-fueled programs are available for your association, school, health care facility, non-profit organization, and business corporation. Dr. Joel Goodman (founder and Director of The Humor Project) and Margie Ingram (Director of Special Programs) have made presentations for more than two million people worldwide. The Speakers Bureau offers over 50 other excellent presenters who provide custom-designed keynote speeches, workshops, and staff development seminars.

"To Life!"
278 Delaware Avenue
Delmar, NY 12054
(518) 439-5975
Fax: (518) 475-9141
www.tolife.org
E-mail: info@ToLife.org

Your personal source for breast cancer education and support.

# Order Form

If you would like to order additional copies of this book, please fill out this order form, and send a check or money order for $14.95, plus $2.50 shipping and handling per book. In New York State, please enclose 7% sales tax on the total order. Please make checks payable to:  HIDDEN HARBOUR PRESS

**NAME:**_____

**ADDRESS:** _____

**CITY:** _____**STATE:** _____

**ZIP:**_____ **E-MAIL:**_____

**NUMBER OF COPIES:** _____

**TOTAL AMOUNT OF ORDER:**_____

**MAIL YOUR ORDERS TO:**

**HIDDEN HARBOUR PRESS**
**P.O. BOX 789**
**SARATOGA SPRINGS, NY**
**12866**

**THANK YOU!**

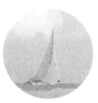

# Postscript

Thanks for taking the time to read all or part of this book. I hope it has been of some help to you—either for coping with your day-to-day crises or, in fact, when the "big one" hit. You've heard all about my "medical odyssey." Do you have any "odysseys" of your own? I'd love to hear about them. Feel free to drop me a line at the address below.

Are you interested in helping your group or organization "keep their boat afloat when the big one hits"? Would you like a keynote speaker for your next conference? Please keep me in mind if you do. I would enjoy meeting you and speaking to your group. I can tailor my talks and workshops to your particular group so they can begin using the tools for handling crises right away.

To contact me by e-mail, write to:

Kjh50@worldnet.att.net

Or you may write to me the old-fashioned way at:

Kim Hupp
P.O. Box 789
Saratoga Springs, NY 12866

Thanks!